# IMMUNITY
# DIET

Also by the author

*The Don't-Diet Plan: A No-Nonsense Guide to Weight Loss*

*Fix It with Food: Superfoods to Become Super Healthy*

*Ultimate Grandmother Hacks:*
*50 Kickass Traditional Habits for a Fitter You*

# The
# IMMUNITY
# DIET

## FIGHT OFF INFECTIONS
### *and* LIVE YOUR BEST LIFE

# KAVITA DEVGAN

RUPA

Published by
Rupa Publications India Pvt. Ltd 2022
7/16, Ansari Road, Daryaganj
New Delhi 110002

*Sales centres:*
Bengaluru Chennai
Hyderabad Jaipur Kathmandu
Kolkata Mumbai Prayagraj

ISBN: 978-93-5520-401-1

Fourth impression 2024

10 9 8 7 6 5 4

The moral right of the author has been asserted.

Printed in India

*To the best gift I ever got—my sister,*
*Punita Mehra*

# Contents

*Foreword by K. Srinath Reddy*     *xi*

*Prologue*     *xiii*

## I
## UNDERSTANDING IMMUNITY

**Facts to Know 1: The Backstory**     **2**

1. What Is Immunity?     3

**Facts to Know 2: The Basics**     **6**

2. The Immunity Warriors     8

## II
## THE LIFESTYLE FIX

**Facts to Know 3: What Makes Our Immunity Strong**     **14**

### *Immunity Boosters*

3. Get Some Sun     17
4. Sleep Well     23
5. Exercise Your Immunity     30
6. Practise Fasting     38
7. Eat Fresh     42
8. Listen to Your Gut     46
9. Do Oil Pulling     52

### *Immunity Downers*

10. Watch Your Weight     57

11. Don't Self-Medicate                                61
12. Keep Inflammation Down                             65
13. Beat the Pollution                                 69

## III
## EAT THE RIGHT FOODS

14. Focus on Fibre                                     79
15. The Spicy Truth                                    82
16. Hydrate Enough                                     87
17. Get the Protein Power                              93
18. Eat Good Fats                                      98
19. The Important Vitamins                            104
20. The Important Minerals                            115
21. The Important Adaptogens                          131
22. The Important Mesonutrients                       140
23. The Essential Nutrient That No One
    Talks About: Enzymes                              153

### *Immunity Downer*

24. Mind the Sugar Attack                             160
**Facts to Know 4: Facts on a Lighter Note**         **165**

## IV
## TAP YOUR MIND

### *Immunity Boosters*

25. Cook Mindfully                                    169
26. Breathe Right                                     174
27. Eat Stress-Free                                   181
28. Tap the Mind Energy                               185
29. Become a Cautious Optimist                        191

*Immunity Downers*

30. Put a Lid on Stress                                    197

**Facts to Know 5: The Memory Connection**            **207**

## V
## COVID-19 AND THE IMMUNITY QUESTION

31. Beating COVID-19 and Its Collateral Damage        211
32. Five Lessons To Learn From COVID-19               222
33. A Simple Post-COVID Diet Care Plan                229

## VI
## TOOLS

34. 50 Immunity Boosters                              235
35. 25 Super Easy Immunity Hacks                      253
36. Recipes                                           255

*Acknowledgements*                                    261

# Foreword

The COVID-19 pandemic has made all of us more aware of the role that our immune system plays in combating infections. We have recognized that a strong immune system can be the vital difference between the contrasting outcomes of an asymptomatic or mildly symptomatic response and severe illness, hospitalization and death when infected by the virus. Scientists have attempted to familiarize us with the nuances of natural innate immunity and acquired immunity that we gain through infection or vaccination. If the virus has played the villain in this long-running drama, the immune system is the intrepid hero that comes to our rescue.

In much of the discourse, the vital role of nutrition received only a passing mention, even as different types of vaccines were extensively described and loudly debated. Yet, if our immune system is our body's defender-in-chief, nutrition is the principal source of its strength and stability. Not only does the immune system function feebly if the body receives inadequate nutrition, but immune mechanisms can go rogue if autoimmunity or inflammation are triggered by inappropriate nutrition. The remarkable array of structures, cells and chemicals that participate and interact dynamically in our immune system is simply amazing. From that complex system, nutrition creates an orchestra that maintains our health in harmony most of the time.

Kavita Devgan decodes the complexity of the immune system for us while providing valuable insights into how we can alter our patterns of daily living and behaviours to enhance our immunity instead of damaging it. She describes how our beliefs and behaviours alter our biology so that we can strengthen our immune system rather than damage it. Nutrition does play a great role, but factors such as sleep and stress also require attention. The book provides the information we can easily assimilate and apply in our daily lives to promote, protect and preserve our health through a well-functioning immune system.

Kavita balances the exactness of scientific information with the elegance of accessible communication to create an engaging book of great value for any reader interested in health. While nutrition is rightly positioned at its heart, the book provides a holistic understanding of how our immune system must be supported and strengthened by the actions that we undertake in our daily lives so that it can protect us at all times with vigilance and vigour.

Professor K. Srinath Reddy
President, Public Health Foundation of India (PHFI)
Former Head of the Department of Cardiology,
All India Institute of Medical Sciences (AIIMS)

Kavita Devgan

# Prologue

If there is one lesson that the testing times of the COVID-19 pandemic have taught us, it is that we need an iron-clad immunity to stay safe and recover faster in case we do get infected. The best news is that it is easily done.

However, at the very outset, we need to understand the fact that we don't 'create' immunity; we just 'build' it. We can prevent its decline and enhance its abilities to ensure that we have a balanced immune system that works at its efficient best.

Fortunately, most of us are born with optimal immunity since our bodies are innately equipped with it. We also acquire immunity to some of the various pathogens we encounter over the course of our lifetime.

As we age, due to environmental assault and our less-than-perfect lifestyles, our immunity first becomes rusty and then slowly gets depleted. That is why it is essential to keep optimizing the functioning of our immune system.

There are enough medical tools inside our body to help prevent diseases and illness, but as these are more often than not severely compromised due to myriad reasons, we need to keep providing assistance to our innate immune system, propping it up with the right habits and cues to keep it relevant, able and effective.

Thankfully our knowledge of the immune system has expanded by volumes over the last few decades. Today we understand how it functions at the cellular and subcellular levels; we know how the system communicates inside the body, how it gets into action, fights and helps purge the unwanted and harmful external intruders. Our understanding of how to strengthen and empower it has also improved. Most importantly, we know that this system is our best and only defence against the unpredictable array of health challenges that we face.

It is evident that we lead lives that undermine this system at every level. So, it is practically mandatory to counteract the diminishing factors simultaneously and continuously, to not just maintain the status quo, but to be able to stay on top of this system for our survival. We also know that while our genes play a huge role in determining our susceptibility to certain diseases, the way we choose to live our everyday lives has the power to influence and change our degree of susceptibility to a considerable extent.

Another significant fact is that immunity can only be strengthened through sustained effort. There are no magic pills, foods or supplements that can deliver immunity overnight or in a short time. We need to work at improving it continuously and diligently, and the only sure-shot way to do so is to lead an immunity-friendly lifestyle and eat immunity-strengthening and foods. There is really no immediate solution or an easy way out.

So, what really is immunity?

Simply put, immunity refers to the ability of our bodies and minds to withstand the stresses of our daily life; it is also the ability to cope with health imbalance and disease. In other words, the body can protect itself from foreign invaders like viruses, disease and infection. We can't feel or see our immunity or take its pulse or its temperature, but our immune system is quietly and constantly patrolling our body to detect and destroy infectious microbes.

Kavita Devgan

The strength of our immune system decides who gets sick and who doesn't—who catches the newest bug in town and who stays fit and fine through the onslaught of new illnesses. And it is this strength that also decides how mild or severe our symptoms are and how fast we recover if we do catch an illness.

Unfortunately, we are progressively becoming people who are immunosuppressed mostly because our lifestyles have undergone a sea change. Over the last few centuries, an average person's lifestyle has undergone a massive transformation— from a healthy diet and exercise-oriented pattern, we have moved to a more sedentary and fast-food-consuming life. This change has led to not just an increase in obesity, but also impaired immunity and led to a scary affinity to infections and lifestyle disorders.

## How to Build Immunity

Certain behavioural changes and a system of smart habits can help us to build our immunity successfully. In this book, I have put together an extensive set of habits that can help boost our immunity, empower this amazingly intelligent system further, and give us an edge to beat whatever the universe throws at us—from everyday injuries, burns, viral infections, bacterial attacks, inflammatory disorders to the yet unseen, new and unfamiliar adversaries.

This list of habits is extensive, and includes the herbs, spices, nutrients and antioxidants we use in everyday cooking, lifestyle factors and our mental state. Adopting certain simple habits can help to not just prevent diseases but also recover effectively as well, thus extending both longevity and the quality of life. Switching to these habits can help us move away from a body that promotes and attracts diseases to a body that actively prevents them and keeps them at bay.

This book is divided into six parts; we begin with understanding the facets of immunity. We then move on to important factors on which our immunity depends—food (nutritional therapy) and lifestyle changes. The significance of our mental health in assisting our immunity cannot be understated, and yet, it is often overlooked. Therefore, we will also discuss our mind matters and how they affect our lifestyles and habits, which in turn, hold the key to the strength of our immunity.

The COVID-19 pandemic has taught us that a strong immunity, robust health and a disease-free life is the best gift we can bestow upon ourselves. Everything else, be it money or exotic holidays or expensive cars, is secondary. To combat the effects of COVID-19 and to best prepare for the uncertainties of the future, this book elaborates on how this virus, that has brought the world to its knees, affects our immunity. And lastly, I hope to equip your disease-fighting arsenal with certain tools, immunity-boosters, hacks and recipes that will help you combat the worst of attacks on your health from foreign intruders.

Let this book be your guide to building a robust and hardy immune system. Read it carefully, as there is no doubt that to best defend against old and new diseases our well-functioning immune system needs regular attention. Consciously building our immunity level is simply a way of taking responsibility for our health and giving our body's inherent healing powers a much-needed fillip.

The essence of the book lies in bringing about a mental shift by which we consciously move away from a mindset of waiting for a disease to happen and then working in overdrive, and exhausting ourselves and our body in trying to defeat it, to an attitude of prevention, where we focus on strengthening our internal healing system consciously and actively. As the adage goes: prevention is better than cure.

I believe that our body and its inherent immunity are precious gifts, but ensuring that it functions at its efficient best, and stay capable of protecting us is our continued responsibility. It is within our power to weaken or strengthen our immune system through the habits we live by. We are given one body for this life, and our continuous aim should be to protect it as it protects us.

# I

## UNDERSTANDING IMMUNITY

## The Backstory

*The earliest known reference to immunity goes back over two millennia. During the plague of Athens in 430 BC, the Greeks realized that people who had survived smallpox didn't contract the disease a second time, and the concept of immunity was born.*

*Before we understood the immune system, doctors diagnosed all illnesses according to the criteria devised by the Greek philosopher Hippocrates—the balance of 'four humours': melancholic, phlegmatic, choleric or sanguine.*

*The key functions of the immune system were discovered by two scientists— Louis Pasteur, a French microbiologist and Robert Koch, a German physician.*

1

# What Is Immunity?

The immune system is an amazing and complex interconnected system of multiple cells, tissues and molecules spread out all over the body. Hundreds of big and small organs, a network of vessels and tissues, billions of specialized cells across our body contribute to our immunity. These immune warriors work towards making our body a fortress and protecting it from billions of parasites, intruders and enemies that may attack us every day.

## Types of Immune Systems

There are two main types of immune systems that work towards the overall functioning of the body and both are equally important in fighting infections—the innate and the specialized adaptive immune system.

The disease resistant fortifications that we are born with form the innate immune system. It is our first line of defence and gets into action merely seconds after an invasion by virus or bacteria. The innate system consists of cells and proteins that are always ready to fight microorganisms at the site of infection and provide general protection, mostly against bacterial infections. Consider it a starter kit that does the heavy lifting and is present at the front of the battle lines. The innate system functions smartly, making important decisions such as determining how dangerous the enemy is and what broad category it falls under. According to the data it collects, it activates the second line of defence, which then falls into action.

The second line of defence is a specialized adaptive immune system that produces a slower response. It contains specialized super cells and antibodies, which coordinate with and support the first line of defence. It gets called into action when pathogens bypass the innate immunity. This system begins as a blank slate at birth, gets powerful with time as one is exposed to pathogens and then, weakens as one ages. It is familiar with all possible intruders, has specific methods to deal with different microorganisms and is equipped with super weapons, the specialized cells to fight them. Both systems are interconnected and their synergy is what makes our immune system so unique and powerful.

A third kind of immunity, called passive immunity, is 'borrowed' from another source and it lasts for a short time. For example, antibodies in breast milk provide newborn babies with temporary immunity against the diseases to which the mother has been exposed, or when a person receives antibodies artificially in the form of an injection (gamma globulin injection).

## The Working

The immune system works by first spotting foreign bacteria, viruses, fungi and parasites hiding in the body, and then sends its troops to destroy the invaders and the tissues they infect. When our border wall is breached, the innate system gets into action. Macrophages followed by the neutrophils, come into play, informed by the cytokines. Complement proteins bring in reinforcements if need be. (Read Chapter 2 to know more about them and how they work.) This is usually enough for mild infections and small wounds.

But if this, too, gets breached, then our adaptive immune system with its specialized cells gets into action. The most powerful weapons in our immune system's arsenal are the white blood cells (WBCs)—comprising lymphocytes, that create antigens for specific pathogens and kill them or escort them out of the body, and phagocytes which ingest harmful bacteria. It is interesting to note that although WBCs account for only 1 per cent of the cells in about 5 litres of blood in an adult's body, there are more than enough cells to get the job done.

## The Basics

*Immunity is a lifelong commitment. There are no shortcuts or permanent solutions; we need to keep augmenting and supporting our body's defence mechanism throughout our lives. The natural age-related deterioration of the immune system is known as immunosenescence.*

*Free radicals are a big threat to our immunity. These are unstable atoms that can damage cells and cause illness. When our body is under oxidative stress due to exposure to UV radiation, air pollution, smoking and drinking alcohol, free radicals are released and they weaken our immune system as they are capable of causing large chain chemical reactions in our body by reacting with other molecules to bring about disease causing changes.*

*Symptoms of a disease are sometimes the result of the immune system doing its job. So there's no need to be scared of a fever or mild inflammation (swelling, redness, pain) as these symptoms indicate that your immune system is working efficiently and fighting the invaders.*

*Our immune system is present throughout our body, with its immune cells working as specialized detectors in all our organs and tissues. The immune system works like the military. There are different branches, each serving a unique function in protecting the body. (Also, see immune warriors.) It is, however, possible for our immune system to malfunction at times. Such malfunction, or reaction to a false alarm, manifests in the form of allergies.*

*The cells in our body are marked with a system called human leukocyte antigen (HLA). These markings inform the immune system that the cells in question are indeed the cells of your body and not a foreign entity that should be attacked. In some cases, the immune system goes into overdrive, gets too* excited and begins attacking normal tissues mistaking them for invaders. This condition is called an autoimmune disease; examples include rheumatoid arthritis, celiac disease and psoriasis.

The immune system, much like the nervous system, is capable of learning. It constantly analyses its experiences, learns from them and passes on the lessons to the future generations of cells.

# The Immunity Warriors

As explained in the last chapter, the immune system is a highly complex system made up of many types of cells and tissues. Let's get introduced to some of its most essential warriors.

## Macrophages

Macrophages are the largest immune cells in the body. Their function within the immune system is to devour dead cells, kill living enemies, coordinate defences and help heal wounds. Their life span ranges from several months to years.

## Neutrophils

When macrophages require help, they send for neutrophils, which assist them in hunting for bacteria. In their fight against pathogens, neutrophils are the self-sacrificing cells. Their life span is very short and they fight only for a few hours.

## Dendritic Cells

These cells function as the messengers and intelligence officers of the immune system. They process data from the samples of the dead intruders and relay the information to the adaptive immune system.

## The Complement System

This army of 30 proteins injure enemies and activate immune cells. They act as superglue and make it easier for immune cells to grab and deactivate their victims.

## Lymphocytes

Lymphocytes are a type of WBC and comprise the bulk of the immune system. There are two types of lymphocytes: B-lymphocytes and T-lymphocytes. Lymphocytes help the body remember the invaders and destroy them in case there are repetitive future attacks.

## Cytokines

These are tiny proteins that are used to convey information. On spotting an invader, T-cells secrete cytokines that activate other immune system cells nearby and attract more immune system cells to the area of the body where they are needed. Simply put, they are the language of our immune cells.

## T-Lymphocytes

T-lymphocytes, also known as T-cells, contain receptors that help them differentiate between the matter that is harmless to the body and that which is dangerous, foreign substance such as virus or bacteria. Once an invader is detected, the different types of T-cells either directly destroy them or assist other immune cells in attacking them. T-cells and macrophages are also called 'killer' cells.

## B-Lymphocytes

Certain cytokines released by T-cells activate and direct another type of lymphocyte, the B-cell, to make specific antibodies against a foreign substance. Each B cell makes a particular type of antibody. For example, there is a specific kind of B cell that helps to fight off the flu. Antibodies then seek the invaders and either neutralize the foreign object directly or mark it for destruction so that other immune cells may finish the task. B-lymphocytes are the body's de facto military intelligence system—they find their targets and send defences to lock onto them.

## The Lymphatic System

Lymph vessels are miles-long, tube-like structures spanning our entire body. They serve as the delivery system for the lymph fluid—a semi-clear liquid that carries water, oxygen and nutrients from the blood system to the cells. The lymph vessels also transport cell waste from the cells and their surroundings to the lymph nodes to be filtered, processed and drained.

The lymph nodes, which serve as a filter for germs, are located all over the body, with the prominent positions being behind the knees and the sides of the neck. These enlarge as they respond to new WBCs produced during infection. So, if you find that your glands are swollen, there's a good chance that your body is trying to fight off an infection. They also contain WBCs, especially lymphocytes, which help fight and track the germs going in and out of the body.

## Spleen

This is a lesser-known organ that lies between the stomach and diaphragm, and its most important function is to manufacture new WBCs and clean out old blood cells from the body. It's also a place where immune cells congregate and convene.

## Tonsils

Located at the back of the throat, tonsils function as bases that actively sample everything that enters the body through the mouth. They train the immune system to differentiate between the harmless food particle and the harmful disease which may find their way along with the food.

## Antibodies

Antibodies are the most specialized arsenal in our immune system. They are disease-specific, highly efficient antigens that attach themselves only to the enemy they are made for, thus helping the immune cells to attack and deactivate them. Additionally, they also serve to activate the complement system.

# II

# THE LIFESTYLE FIX

## What Makes Our Immunity Strong?

*Weakened immunity is most commonly found in people and communities with high nutrient gaps and deficiencies, specifically of vitamins A, B6, C, D3 and E, alongside other micronutrients such as selenium and zinc, and very often, protein too. These nutrient gaps must be addressed for an effective immune system.*

*Avoiding all germs is not suitable for the immune system. Living in an overly sterile environment reduces the risk of these pathogens entering the human body. This can result in a weakened immune system because it does not get a chance to be primed against different kinds of microbes and organisms, and its growth is impaired. So, it is advisable to practise good hygiene, but it is best not to go overboard.*

*During extremely hectic and frantically busy times, if you suddenly fall sick, consider it a sign from your immune system. Not sleeping enough can affect your immune system and leave you susceptible to cold, flu and infection. There is a steep increase in the levels of melatonin in our blood during sleep, which is a known immunity booster. So, sleep enough and sleep well every day.*

*Regular exercise changes brain chemistry and leads to the release of beta-endorphins in the brain, which cut depression, increase the feeling of accomplishment and create general well-being and optimism. Exercise-induced positive immune system changes are short-lived; they last for a few hours to a day. One must exercise regularly to score these benefits. However, too much exercise is not a good idea, as there is a connection between overtraining and increased susceptibility to infections. A stressful event can depress our immune system for up to 24 hours. In the long run, trauma, sadness and anger can* substantially reduce immunity, so it is vital to address these issues and come to terms with them through counselling, support groups or writing therapy. Similarly, a pleasant and uplifting experience, such as going out for a meal with friends, watching a nice movie or enjoying a good meal can strengthen our immune system for as long as two days. So, consciously make time for happy moments.

Staying out of harm's way is essential for the health of our immune system. Excessive consumption of alcohol, marijuana, cocaine, tobacco, environmental toxins, antibiotics or ultraviolet (UV) rays can impair immunity, so it is best to steer clear of them.

Our daily diet is perhaps the most significant factor that affects our immunity. It is also the one factor to which we can make incremental changes every day for a strong body and immunity. Maintain a balance between carbohydrate and protein intake as both are essential macronutrients. Carbohydrates stimulate the release of a neurochemical called serotonin in the brain that calms anxiety and creates a feeling of well-being and peace. Meals rich in animal protein increase dopamine and norepinephrine, which are compounds that heighten alertness, focus and aggression. We need a good balance of both kinds of emotions to feel well.

# IMMUNITY BOOSTERS

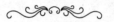

3

# Get Some Sun

I have a morning ritual. I do surya namaskar, make an offering of water to the sun in prayer and only then do I have my breakfast in the balcony, sitting facing the sun. My best friend has her morning and evening cup of tea sitting under the sun in her balcony as well. My mother's date with the sun happens mid-morning when she tends to her plants, and my cousin tries not to miss his 30-minute walk during his lunch hour.

When did you last say hello to the sun?

## Why Do You Need the Sun?

Soaking in some sunlight is a scientifically proven solution to score enough vitamin D—an essential fat-soluble vitamin that is important for cell growth. Our body produces vitamin D when our skin is exposed to sunlight.

Sunlight helps warm both our body and the soul, and the sunniest news of all is that the divine rays of the sun will keep you slimmer too! That's because the vitamin D our body produces when exposed to sunlight directly relates to our metabolism and, thus, how much we weigh. And it goes without saying that sunlight is an instant mood booster on a gloomy, grey day. Our bodies also use vitamin D to absorb and maintain healthy levels of calcium and phosphorus, both of which are important to grow and strengthen our bones. It also helps reduce inflammation in the body and boosts our immunity.

A deficiency of vitamin D, besides leading to an increase in our weight, can also cause body aches and pains, an increased risk for rickets (softening and weakening of bones in children), osteoporosis (weak and brittle bones), cardiovascular diseases, diabetes, cancer and infections such as tuberculosis, besides lowering immunity immensely.

## The Flip Side

Too much exposure to UV radiation can suppress the immune system's response to bacterial, viral and fungal infections. So while too much exposure may be a bad idea, we do need some sun on our skin to stay safe and healthy.

## The Immunity Connection

Vitamin D helps keep the immune system balanced and its deficiency increases our susceptibility to infections. It is essential to modulate both kinds of immune systems in our body—the innate system that fights infections quickly and the adaptive system (See Chapter 1 for more details) responsible for the production of antibodies.

How our body responds to infection is dependent on the levels of vitamin D in our body. Many cells in the body, including immune cells, such as WBCs, contain vitamin D receptors and activating enzymes on their surface. Vitamin D helps strengthen the function of immune cells such as T-cells and macrophages, which affects how these cells multiply and mature into active cells. Since T-cells do not mobilize if they detect only small amounts of vitamin D in the bloodstream, healthy levels of this vitamin lead to a greater number of T-cells being present at the site of infection. (Flip to Chapter 2 to know more.)

Additionally, vitamin D induces the production of anti-microbial peptides in the skin; these compounds help defend the body against new infections. Low vitamin D levels are associated with an increased risk of respiratory diseases, including tuberculosis, asthma, chronic obstructive pulmonary disease (COPD), viral and bacterial infections. A deficiency could also lead to decreased lung function, directly affecting our body's ability to fight respiratory infections.

Finally, vitamin D and magnesium, both essential immunity-boosting nutrients, are dependent on each other for their efficiency since the former helps stimulate the absorption of the latter in the body. So we see that vitamin D, apart from the myriad benefits, is also essential in harnessing magnesium's immunity-boosting effect.

## The Vitamin D Irony

For a hot, tropical country that receives ample sunlight throughout the year, it is surprising how much of our population suffers from a deficiency of vitamin D. In fact, in my wellness and diet counselling sessions, I've noticed a common trend of vitamin D deficiency in most of my clients.

## Why Is It So Rampant?

There are many reasons for this rampant deficiency, the most important being that we simply don't spend enough time outdoors in sunlight. Most of our waking hours are spent inside the house or office. Our indoor lifestyle in air-conditioned homes and workplaces with screens that block sunlight everywhere, including in cars, does not allow our skin to get adequate sun exposure to make necessary vitamin D.

Secondly, most Indians are blessed with melanin-rich, dark skin. Melanin, an innate skin pigment, acts as a natural sunblock and absorbs the sun's UV rays to help protect the skin against damage from excess sunlight. Therefore, Indians need to spend longer in the sun to produce the same amount of vitamin D.

An important factor in the widespread vitamin D deficiency is the lack of access to vitamin D fortified foods. The limited sources of this elusive vitamin, namely egg yolk and fatty fish (salmon, sardines, tuna and mackerel) are not viable options for vegetarians. Mushrooms are the only vegetarian food with substantial levels of vitamin D. It is also important to note that simply adding vitamin D to our diet is not enough to prevent deficiency.

### Good to Know

Vitamin D levels can be measured with a simple blood test. For a strong immune system, we should aim to maintain 50–60 ng/ml of vitamin D in our blood.

## The Bottom Line

Regular sun exposure (without sunscreen on our skin) is the best way to get enough vitamin D. So, my strong suggestion is that you rack up some sunlight-filled hours every week, look closely at your plate, and if the levels have still not improved, opt for a supplement. This vitamin is too essential to the health of our immunity and general well-being to ignore it or leave it to chance.

# TO-DO

To get enough vitamin D:

- Try to step out for 15–20 minutes during the sunniest hour of the day (anytime between 10.00 a.m. to 2.00 p.m.). You can make it a ritual to take a short walk after lunch. Or walk your pet around the block in the morning. Regular walk in the sun will not only lead to an increase in vitamin D, but will also help burn calories.
- Eat whole eggs (with the yolk) for breakfast. If you are a vegetarian, breakfast cereal or instant oats fortified with vitamin D3 are a healthy, plant-based alternative. Often milk and even non-dairy options like soy and almond milk are also fortified with vitamin D. Make sure you read the labels carefully and shop wisely.
- Include salmon or tuna or sautéed mushrooms in at least one meal every day.
- Vitamin D is stored in the body for approximately two months. Therefore, the stock of vitamin D replenished during the sunny summer days starts depleting during the shorter and colder days in the winter. So don't forget to take your vitamin D supplement when the days start getting chilly.
- Today, for most people, vitamin D is no longer an optional supplement but has become a cellular necessity. Anyone above the age of four should have 10 micrograms of vitamin D (400 IU) daily, particularly during the winter months. People at higher risk (those with little or no exposure to the sun and people with dark skin) are advised to take a supplement all year round.

*Tip: Be aware that vitamin D supplements, taken over a very long period, can cause calcium build-up that can weaken the bones and damage the kidneys and the heart. So, you must keep a check on your levels through regular tests.*

- Choose the supplement wisely.
  - Opt for vitamin D3 (cholecalciferol) supplement rather than vitamin D2 (ergocalciferol or pre-vitamin D) as the former is better absorbed and is more efficient at increasing vitamin D levels in the body.
  - If you are vegan, then check the label on vitamin D3 supplements to make sure they are derived from lichen (symbiotic life form of fungi and algae) rather than lanolin, a waxy substance that comes from sheep's wool.
  - Know that taking the supplement daily or weekly is more effective than larger doses taken as monthly doses. Since vitamin D is a fat-soluble vitamin, it need not be taken every day and can be taken once every seven to 15 days.

**Fun Fact:** Vitamin D is the only vitamin our body produces and it's actually a hormone!

# 4

# Sleep Well

Are you someone who loves to boast about the all-nighters you pull? Do you brag that you can get by with very little sleep, sometimes no sleep at all? Do you, like my neighbour, love to flaunt the fact that you just cannot sleep before 3 a.m.? You'd be surprised to learn what you're depriving your body of by not sleeping enough.

## Why Do You Need Sleep?

Groggy mornings and dragging yourself through the day after staying awake till late the previous night is proof that you are your best self only when you're well-rested. A good night's sleep makes you a more efficient and mentally-present individual who can take whatever life throws their way head-on, and that includes the various pathogens we encounter every single day. Yes, your immune system is at its best only after a night of quality sleep.

Dark circles under the eyes, low energy and fatigue are all tell-tale signs of a wrong sleeping pattern, but the damage runs deeper. Chronic sleep deprivation can result in health issues like diabetes, hormonal imbalances, memory loss, high blood pressure, heart problems, weight gain, lower sexual drive, depression and more, besides, of course, completely derailing our immunity.

## The Immunity Connection

The connection of sleep with immunity is actually very straightforward—optimal immune function requires adequate sleep and inadequate sleep impairs the immune response. In fact, not getting enough sound sleep can negatively impact stress levels, immune function and disease resistance. Our immune system is the best defence against catching a disease, and not sleeping enough can reduce its strength and functionality and wear it down severely.

When we are asleep, our immune system, along with our brain and other body processes, is still hard at work and conducts repairs and rejuvenates our body and mind. Sleep time gives our body's internal handymen a chance to fix whatever is wrong. Therefore, not sleeping well leads to an unprepared immune system that has not had time to work on the wear and tear in your body during the day, thus making you a little more susceptible to pathogens than you normally would be.

Lack of sleep also decreases the production of cytokines, a type of protein that fights infection and inflammation. Sound sleep improves the functioning of other immune cells such as T-cells. In fact, poor sleep may lead to stress hormones inhibiting the ability of T-cells to function effectively. Finally, sleep helps the brain form memories, even immune memories (See Chapter 2).

These important immune memories are formed by our endocrine system during deep, non-rapid-eye-movement sleep. Vaccines rely on those immunological memories to work correctly. Vaccinations work to help the body build an antibody response so that when the pathogen you are vaccinated against tries to attack, the body remembers and responds effectively. This kind of long-term memory gets strengthened by sleep—and suppressed by loss of sleep.

**Good to Know**

The optimal amount of sleep for most adults varies, but often seven to eight hours (of good sleep) each night is a universal benchmark. Teenagers may need nine to 10 hours of sleep, with school going children needing about 10 or more hours of sleep.

---

## TO-DO

### Food Solutions

- Eat your last meal at least two to three hours before bedtime to let your body get into rest mode. If the last meal of the day is just before your sleeping time, this process gets hampered.

- If you eat very little all day and gorge at night, it's time to change that. Keep dinner light and eat easily digestible foods. Dinners high in fats prove to be heavy on your digestive system, and all the gas production and consequent rumblings in your stomach may keep you awake, grumbling and uneasy. Similarly, highly seasoned and spicy food may also interfere with sleep, especially if one is prone to heartburn. Going to bed when you can't eat another bite revs up the body systems, particularly the digestive system; even though you may feel drowsy and fall asleep quicker after a heavy meal, all the intestinal machinations needed to digest a large-sized meal may lead to frequent waking and a relatively poor quality of sleep. So, it is best to keep your dinner light—khichdi, a combination of rice and dal (lentils), is a wonderful, easily-digestible and sleep-inducing food.

- Your sleeping posture matters just as much when it comes

to sleep quality. Sleeping on a distended belly filled with food pushes the stomach and the diaphragm upwards, compressing the space for the lungs, which may cause trouble in breathing during the night.

- 'Waker' foods keep us awake by stimulating the neurochemicals that perk up the brain. So it is wise to be wary of too much caffeine—strong coffee or cola or 'energy' drinks—late in the day. Caffeine is a stimulant and accelerates not only the nervous system, but may also cause an increase in adrenaline in our blood which sets off an increase in breathing rate, heart rate, urine output and the production of stomach acids. Your body working in overdrive when you want to slow things down is not conducive to a restful sleep. Even small amounts of caffeine can affect your sleep, especially if you are sensitive to caffeine. To prepare your body for deep and relaxing sleep, avoid drinking caffeine-rich beverages like tea, coffee or sports drinks and eating foods like chocolates four to six hours before bedtime.

- Alcohol may seem the quickest way to get knocked out and hit the sack. However, it seriously impairs the quality of sleep. Alcohol-induced blackout may result in an unconscious state for the first two to three hours, but this will, more often than not, be followed by disturbed sleep, frequent urination and dehydration. You will also end up waking up tired and hungover. Alcohol and other similar depressants suppress rapid eye movement (REM) sleep, the phase of sleep during which one experiences dreaming. A shorter REM stage makes for night awakenings and restless sleep.

*Tip: Don't drink any alcohol within two hours of bedtime. And, of course, never mix alcohol with sleeping pills or any other medication as alcohol can change how a medication works and can cause trouble.*

- A key to a restful night's sleep is to calm our minds down after the hustle and bustle of the day. 'Sleeper' foods contain tryptophan, an amino acid that helps our body produce sleep-inducing chemicals like serotonin and melatonin. Now let's look at a few snooze foods, high in the sleep-inducing amino acid tryptophan:

  - Dairy products such as cottage cheese, cheese, milk
  - Soy products such as soy milk, tofu, soybean nuts
  - Seafood
  - Meats
  - Poultry
  - Whole grains: bajra, barley, millets
  - Beans
  - Rice
  - Hummus
  - Lentils
  - Hazelnuts, Peanuts
  - Eggs
  - Sesame seeds, sunflower seeds
  - Colocassia
  - Sweet Potato
  - Cashew nuts
  - Mango

*Tip: Munching on a couple walnuts before bedtime will help raise melatonin, a hormone that regulates night and day cycles or sleep-wake cycles in the body.*

- A blanket ban on carbohydrates in your dinner won't offer much relief, as carbohydrates make the amino acid tryptophan more available to the brain. A carbohydrate-rich meal stimulates the release of insulin (the fat storage and blood sugar regulating hormone), which helps clear other amino acids that compete with tryptophan in the bloodstream, allowing more of this natural sleep-inducing amino acid to enter the brain and produce sleep-inducing chemicals. In fact, eating a high-protein meal without accompanying carbohydrates may, in fact, keep you awake, since protein-rich foods contain the amino acid tyrosine, which perks up the brain.

## Other Solutions

- If it is stress keeping you awake, then it may help to develop sleep rituals such as listening to relaxing music, reading, journaling, having a cup of warm milk or doing relaxation exercises.

*Tip: A hot bath 60 minutes before bedtime helps relax the body, making you feel sleepy.*

- Overstimulation in the form of revving your mind up with video games, movies or other activities, particularly in front of screens, can disrupt the natural sleep cycle, reduce the amount of melatonin the body is producing and severely increase your insomnia. You'll find yourself frustrated, tossing and turning in bed and not being able to sleep, which will lead to a vicious cycle of overstimulation and sleepless nights. The solution here is simple—limit screen time before bedtime.
- Do you see sleep as a luxury, either due to your personality type (competitive, type A) or due to external pressures from the competitive society? Here, the solution lies in

setting boundaries—both internally and externally and making sleep a priority.

**Fun Fact:** According to an old Irish proverb, 'a good laugh and a long sleep are the best cures in the doctor's book'.

5

# Exercise Your Immunity

My friend's grandfather had told me long ago, 'What they call trekking is our daily routine'. He and his friends used to go for a walk every morning for an hour, and he told me that they did not consider it exercise; instead, what they did in that hour was a seamless part of their daily plan, as important as any other activity they'd do in the course of the day. 'It's as natural for us as eating or sleeping,' he told me. I shared this anecdote in my book, Ultimate Grandmother Hacks, and I am sharing it here again because it elucidates the importance of exercise ever so clearly.

## Why Do You Need to Exercise?

It'll come as no surprise that regular exercise helps the cardiovascular system, improves blood flow, flushes away toxins from muscles and helps keep the kidneys and endocrine system working well. It also helps remove germs and circulate antibodies. All these benefits can help create a fitter, healthier you. Exercise can give us toned limbs and a strong physique, but if you are exercising just to burn calories and get thinner, then you are taking the wrong road. In order to achieve that goal, you need to alter your diet as well.

That said, before you go and cancel your gym membership, give away your running shoes or make that drawing room couch your home, please know that regular exercise can actually help enhance your immunity immensely. In fact, at the first sneeze, it is better if people reach for walking shoes, since exercise is proven to be the best thing one can do to boost their body's immune system and keep the bugs at bay.

## The Immunity Connection

Exercise actually helps strengthen all three layers of our immune system. Those who exercise regularly have often observed that their skin heals faster after wounds and this helps reduce the risk of entry of the bacteria and virus. Our skin is our first line of defence. If the pathogen somehow gains entry, our innate (or natural) immunity that comprises immune cells like neutrophils and natural killer cells comes into play. When we exercise, our muscles contract, the flow of blood and lymph to these muscles increases and immune cells move into the bloodstream at a higher rate. Then, they traverse the body, seek out pathogens and damaged cells and wipe them out. Exercise keeps our immune system's surveillance activity (when immune cells are in the bloodstream looking for infection) active and effective. As discussed earlier, our immunity tends to weaken as we age, therefore, the third line of defence which is the adaptive (or memory) immunity, made of T-lymphocytes and B-lymphocytes can only be maintained in a high count with regular exercise.

There's more!

When we are physically active, our lungs work harder to supply the additional oxygen that our muscles need. This extra work helps us use our lungs to their fullest capacity and makes them stronger. In addition, regular exercise may even help the lungs to rid themselves of airborne viruses and bacteria that are associated with respiratory tract infections.

Working out helps reduce inflammation, which is extremely beneficial as the efficiency of our immunity comes down drastically if our body is inflamed. Cytokines are produced when our muscles contract during exercise. One of these cytokines, IL-6, initially promotes inflammation (an important first response of the immune system against infection), but is shortly followed by an increase in anti-inflammatory cytokines.

Finally, exercise helps us stay happy, and the more stress free and happier we are, the better our immunity is. This connection in fact is very strong. First, dopamine (a neurotransmitter that keeps us happy) in our brain needs to be replenished regularly and the best way to increase its production is by exercising regularly. Second, exercise helps to provide an outlet for nervous energy, take our mind off of our everyday stresses (at least momentarily) and improves our body image. Third, exercise helps reduce the outflow of stress-related hormones that suppress the immune system. Finally, exercise also releases endorphins, those feel-good hormones that improve our sleep quality and cut stress levels—two known components that can compromise the immune system. It's a fact that you score a more restful sleep when you exercise.

*Tip: The key to restful slumber may be as simple as going for a brisk walk (or some other exercise) four to five days a week.*

### Good to Know
The immune-boosting effects of exercise are fairly
short-lived, so the key is to exercise regularly.
You can't exercise once in a while and
hope to create iron-clad immunity.

There is a cumulative effect at play
and the benefits add up as time goes on,
something that will eventually go away
if you don't work out consistently.

## The Flip Side

When we talk of exercise, there's a fine line between healthy, balanced and overdoing it. Overtraining can lead to excess fatigue and mood disturbances, and thus increase inflammation and weaken the immune system. So, keep the intensity of your exercise moderate to high so as to give sufficient stimulus to push the immune cells into circulation. But avoid severe, muscle-damaging workouts as the muscle repair process may actually compete with your immune function and may even put you in a stressful state leading to immune system dysfunction that can last anywhere from a few hours to a few days.

*Tip: Don't overdo it—30–60 minutes of exercise five times a week is considered optimum and sufficient to accrue health benefits for most people.*

---

### TO-DO

It is critical that you take out at least half an hour of every day for exercise because it enhances the other 23.5 hours of your day. Here are some tips that might help:

- Make physical activity a priority. Write it into your schedule and then stick to it.
- Remember to not give in to self-made excuses. Keep responses ready for every possible excuse.

- Consciously make time for exercise. Get up half an hour earlier, walk during the lunch hour, or turn off the television in the evening and step out instead.
- Exercise throughout the day; walk up the stairs instead of taking the elevator, walk to the restaurant instead of taking a cab, walk round the block after lunch, clean your car every morning, thoroughly dust and clean one room in the house every day, rearrange your wardrobe and so on.
- Keep in mind the 21-day rule—if you stick with something for 21 days, it becomes a habit. Keep a journal for the 21 days or mark it off on a calendar. Before you know it, exercise and activity will become a habit.
- An exercise routine doesn't have to be boring and dull. The best exercise is your favourite exercise. Think fun and try a variety of workouts because repetitive workouts every day of the week might not be your cup of tea.
- A variety of exercises will help you stick with the routine— take a long walk twice a week, do aerobics every alternate day and play your favourite outdoor sport on the weekend.
- Keep yourself motivated by writing out your goals and putting them up in a place where you can't ignore them, like the fridge. Maintaining an exercise journal will help you realize and actualize your goals.
- Surround yourself with people who are physically active. If you see other people exercising in the neighbourhood, you will feel like exercising as well.
- You can even try to find a diet or exercise buddy or ask for a friend's help. This will make it easier to stay focused on your goal of a healthier lifestyle.
- Look for simple things you can change about your lifestyle to increase physical activity. This may mean walking around the block while your child is at piano practice or

briskly walking up and down the stairs during lunch hour, spending 15 minutes every evening at home to weed the garden or vacuuming the house every other day and so on.

- Be creative. Maybe get together with friends for a marathon walk-and-talk once or twice a week or fix up a bicycle race for every Saturday morning.
- Your workout doesn't have to take a lot of time. Even half an hour of working out diligently pays off. Can't cram your sweat session into one 30-minute stretch? Fret not! You can also do it in three 10-minute bursts throughout the day as that is just as effective at clearing fat from the bloodstream as exercising continuously for 30 minutes. Be flexible! In fact, look at it this way: even if you do three minutes every hour in a 10-hour period, you've done 30 minutes. And something is always better than nothing.
- Don't shy away from asking for help. Discuss your exercise programme with your doctor before you start. Enlist the services of fitness experts. They can help tailor your exercise programme to be the best 'fit' for you.
- Look for opportunities to do non-structured exercises. You can burn calories just by increasing the intensity of everyday activities too. For example, you can play hide and seek with your children or take the dog for a run.
- Set fitness goals. Commit to walking or running a certain distance in one month, three months or six months. Work on increasing the number of laps you swim each day.
- Don't beat yourself up if you skip a day or two. The important thing is that you get back to it and fast.
- Make fluid intake a part of your workout routine to avoid dehydration. Look out for the warning signs—muscle cramps, dizziness, light-headedness, nausea and headache.
- When you are exercising, don't just think muscles, think

mind too. Swap your treadmill for the leafy avenue to get more well-rounded benefits. When you exercise outdoors, not only do you burn calories and increase muscle power, but also score an all-round sense of well-being. Exposure to nature helps decrease the blood pressure and reduces stress, and you get an optimum dose of vitamin D as well.

**Fun Fact:** Did you know that gardening actually burns more calories than walking the treadmill? Need more incentive? No membership fees is required and you get your daily dose of vitamin D naturally.

- Want a workout that returns maximum value in minimum time? There's nothing better than climbing stairs. The vertical component involved here increases the benefits (read calorie expense), compared to other regular exercises like walking or even jogging. It is also a good cross-training activity because it gets the heart and lungs pumping hard.
- Sitting down all day may actually negate the benefit of your pulse quickening workouts. So along with regular exercise, avoid sitting in one place for too long. Take that five-minute break from your desk job every now and then and walk around a bit.
- Try to exercise in the morning, as this helps get the workout done and out of the way early in the day. Second, as endorphins kick in, your stress levels throughout the day will be regulated. Third, the overnight fast will force the body to burn body fat for energy which will reflect on the scale and on your waist. Finally, working out first thing in the morning revs up the metabolism, which then stays elevated throughout the day, helping you burn more

calories and lose more weight. If you work out in the evening you may still burn fat, but as soon as you go to sleep, your metabolism will slow down and you'll miss out on all the extra fat that you could have burned during the day considering the alternative.

- Go micro. Small, micro-workouts, which are essentially high intensity but brief workouts, may be better for our health than low intensity and continuous exercises.

- Avoid exercising in extreme weather conditions because the changes that are required to help regulate the body's temperature can be stressful to the immune response. So, during cold weather (winter months) plan more indoor activities like stationary biking or walking or jogging on a treadmill. During the summer months finish your outdoor physical activities earlier in the morning or later in the evening to escape the heat of the day.

- Finally, don't push yourself to exercise if you aren't feeling well. When you are unwell, the immune system is already under strain trying to fight the infection. The related stress caused by exercise may challenge recovery.

**Fun Fact:** We use 200 muscles to take a single step forward.

# 6

# Practise Fasting

My friend's naani (maternal grandmother) fasts three times a week, my naani fasted every Monday. My mausi (maternal aunt) fasts on special religious days like poornamashi, Shivratri, navratras, etc. I don't fast for religious reasons, but do it when I feel the need for it, sometimes for two days at a stretch. Whatever the cause or justification, fasting has been a part of our way of living for a long time now and for a good reason.

## Why Do You Need to Practise Fasting?

What is fasting? Fasting is a discipline where one willingly gives their body and digestive system a break by not eating solid food for a certain period of time.

Our bodies are programmed to withstand periods of fasting. Fasting helps redirect energy towards healing and repairing. From weight loss to reversing ageing, improved fitness and superior cognitive abilities to better lipid profile and lowered blood sugar levels—the benefits are immense.

Fasting actually works like a cleaning process, clearing damage and helping remove the cellular junk that can lead to excess weight, wrinkles and myriad diseases. That is why it has become a top health hack in the recent years. We don't need any special equipment or a manual. While fasting is a good option for losing weight, it is an even more effective and brilliant tool for boosting our immunity.

## The Modus Operandi

Fasting or time restricted feeding, which is commonly known as intermittent fasting, is known to regulate our body's glucose, lipid metabolism and the circadian clock (sleep clock). It accelerates DNA repair and boosts the immune system and cognitive function. Fasting has been found to be a protective measure against cancer, obesity, diabetes, metabolic syndrome, inflammation, Alzheimer's disease and several neuropsychiatric disorders. Plus, it is associated with better cardiovascular health, endurance, lower blood pressure and reduced inflammation in the body. In fact, fasting improves every aspect of our health—physical, mental, emotional, intellectual as well as spiritual.

## The Immunity Connection

The positive changes mentioned in the last section help reset our immune system and make it stronger. When you starve, the system tries to save energy and to do so it recycles a lot of immune cells that are not needed, especially those that may be damaged. Fasting gives our digestive system a break and lets the body work on strengthening immunity and other body systems instead. It helps the body cleanse itself, and repair and rejuvenate the cells.

A big benefit of fasting is the activation of autophagy in the body. Autophagy involves cellular pruning, recycling of old, damaged and unwanted cells, and this leads to the production of new cells that are superior in function. As part of the process, autophagy causes the count of the WBCs to drop since the defective ones are eliminated. This triggers the production of new, more effective WBCs. Fasting creates sustained energy deficits, which are the primary triggers for autophagy. Fasting, in fact, can help in renewing, repairing and rejuvenating our entire immune system and thus make it more efficient and robust.

### Good to Know

Other ways to trigger autophagy include exercising, consuming specific nutrients and compounds in healthy, antioxidant-rich foods like curcumin (turmeric), going into controlled ketosis, along with adequate sleep.

---

### TO-DO

- The rules of fasting are flexible. It's not a punishment and can actually be enjoyable if one follows a safe, healthy pattern that works for them. Here are a few options to choose from:
  - Fasting 10 hours for seven days a week
  - Fasting 16 hours for two days a week
  - A juice or a fruit cleanse, one day a week
  - You can find your own fasting schedule and even choose what foods are permitted during your fast— only fruit, raw fruits and vegetables, only lentils, grains once a day, eating before sunset and so on.
- Those who are trained at fasting and do so regularly, can even extend their fasting time from 18 to 20 hours. If you'd like to be able to do the same, start with a shorter duration and with time, increase your tolerance. It is essential that you listen to your body; if you experience

any dizziness, diarrhoea, headache or stomach pain take it as an indication that it's time to break your fast.

- Always break the fast with a low carbohydrate, high protein and moderate fat meal. This will prevent the insulin level from skyrocketing.
- Take as many walks as possible on the days you are fasting. Exercise is a trigger for autophagy and will help to ramp up the fat burning process.
- You can drink coffee during the fast since it gives a healthy boost to autophagy. Decaffinated coffee works just as well.

### Good to Know
The idea behind fasting is not to begin starving yourself, as that will only be counterproductive to your goal, but stop the overeating.

**Fun Fact:** In 2016, the Nobel Prize for Physiology or Medicine was awarded to Dr Yoshinori Ohsumi for unravelling cellular mechanisms of autophagy in humans.

# 7

# Eat Fresh

My mom's bags are always full of seeds for vegetables that she wants to try growing at home, never mind if they are too exotic or delicate for the extreme weather conditions in her part of the world. She gets them, labours over them and often succeeds. Her success tastes sweet.

A close friend of mine gets up early every Sunday to go to the farmers' market and spend her morning stocking up on the freshest, healthiest produce. She buys all her produce only from the farmers' market. A colleague frets about her balcony herb garden like people would for their pets when going away on a vacation.

They all tell me that once you've tasted the freshness of home-grown fruit, vegetables and herbs, you get hooked for life. The flavour and quality of home-grown food is far superior to anything you can buy in a supermarket.

## Why Do You Need to Eat Fresh?

For starters, fresh produce from a farm, be it big or small (whether in the suburbs or your balcony garden) tastes different; it tastes more wholesome. If you've grown the food yourself, you know exactly what you've put into it, you can be sure that it's free from any harmful pesticides and chemicals. Not everyone can grow food or have access to farmers' market. But everyone can try to buy locally-grown fresh produce.

## The Immunity Connection

The sooner you eat a fruit or vegetable after it's picked, the better it is for you nutritionally. Research has proven that the lesser the time lapse between plucking veggies and fruit and eating them, the higher the nutrient composition of that food will be. As time passes, produce loses some of its nutritional value and it is absolutely clear that eating enough nutrients is a prerequisite for good, robust immunity, and deficiencies of the same can be a big immunity downer.

So, when you eat fresh food plucked off the branch or pulled from the earth—bursting with goodness, nutrients, antioxidants and enzymes—there can be no doubt about the value component of these nutritionally dense foods.

It is important to note that the vegetables that are allowed to ripen on the plant will have more nutrients compared to those that are picked early and ripen in storage.

**Good to Know**
Frozen vegetables are often just as healthy as fresh ones because they are usually blanched and frozen immediately, right out of the farm.

It is noteworthy that, during the pandemic, the uncertainty around the food system and access to fresh food brought forth the importance of keeping the food chain (at least the basic needs) as close to us as possible. One lesson we have all learnt during the pandemic is the importance of keeping as less physical distance as possible between source and consumption point.

Finally, eating fresh takes the food from ordinary to extraordinary; it satisfies cravings, nourishes and delights us. It doesn't really take that much to grow or source fresh produce.

It just takes some awareness and willingness. Make a decision to only eat fresh and stick to it. Every small beginning counts, considering the huge payback.

---

## TO-DO

- Take cues from a colleague's herb garden and start work on your kitchen garden, begin accompanying neighbours to the Sunday Farmer's Markets, borrow some exotic (or otherwise) seeds from friends which can be grown at home. Start small, but start today.

- The biggest excuse (and quite a valid one), is space, or rather the lack of it. It is a fact that not all of us have gardens to potter about in, but usually we all do have a balcony or two that we can make use of. You don't really need a lot of ground space to create wonders with, even a small space can be used constructively to grow enough for a small family.

- Don't even have a spare balcony? How about putting your kitchen windowsill to use and grow herbs that are used in your kitchen every day? Everyone has room for a small pot of rosemary, thyme, basil or mint. In fact, if not in the kitchen, any sunny windowsill will do. So, you can start with herbs as they are very easy to grow. Herbs enhance the taste and texture of almost anything. Just compare the cost of a modest herb garden with that of commercially bought small packets and you'll know why this is a brilliant idea. No more bargaining with vendors for free dhaniya (coriander) or green chillies while shopping for vegetables, just grow your own!

- Other easy foods to grow are onions, garlic, chillies, tomatoes, potatoes, leafy greens like lettuce and spinach. Imagine plucking fresh salad greens minutes before you eat them for lunch, or deciding between okra and brinjals from your very own mini-farm to cook for dinner.

- If you have a wall or railing that faces the sun and you'd like to beautify it, consider growing vertical crops such as peas and cucumbers. A hanging basket of cherry tomato vines won't just look good, it'll also supply your salad.

**Fun Fact:** Growing fruits and veggies at home will make your space look lush, green and beautiful as well.

8

# Listen to Your Gut

When people come to me for consultations, I talk about getting their gut back in order first. And this strategy always works. It nets them relief from whatever issue they are facing—high blood sugar, hypertension, fatty liver, obesity and, as a bonus, also sets them on a healthier path for life by strengthening their immunity.

Do you know how much of our immune system lies in our gut? Almost 70 per cent. Yes, that is why a healthy gut is the cornerstone of a healthy immune system.

## Why Do You Need to Listen to Your Gut?

A diseased, gastric system doesn't just lead to multiple gastric troubles, ranging from loose motions to constipation and more, it is bad news for our immunity too. In fact, keeping our gut happy is imperative for keeping sickness at bay. It's simple; a healthy gut means you will:

- have more energy everyday
- fall sick less often
- recover quickly from sickness
- have more mental clarity
- be emotionally stronger

An unhealthy gut often translates to:

- autoimmune diseases
- diabetes
- emotional distress (anxiety, depression)
- neurological issues like Alzheimer's, autism, attention-deficit/hyperactivity disorder

## The Modus Operandi

We are more bacteria than we are human. Yes, there are more bacterial cells—approximately 38 trillion on an average—than human cells in our body. These bacteria live on the skin, in the nose and ears, but largely in our gut. The ecosystem of bacteria in our gut, called the microbiota, is very diverse; there are thousands of species, all with different functions, doing a staggering number of functions crucial for our health. They protect us from infections, shape and boost our immune system, digest the food we eat, and help make and absorb vital nutrients that our body needs for surviving.

Now let's get down to the good, the bad and the ugly. There are good bacteria and bad bacteria present in our gut, and our equation with the two is simple—when the balance is tilted in the favour of the good bacteria, it ensures good health. So, the smart thing to do is to befriend the good guys, choose them wisely and ensure that more of these are produced in the gut to tilt the balance in their favour. Unfortunately, our lifestyles are rife with stress, junk food, antibiotics, pollution etc., all of which kill the good bacteria and tilt the balance in the favour of the bad bacteria. Maintaining this balance, therefore, requires constant effort on our part. It needs a diet that can help keep up the number of good bacteria, so that the net stays positive.

## The Immunity Connection

Healthy bacteria in the gut stimulate the development of T-cells, which, as discussed in earlier chapters, help distinguish between foreign pathogen and our body's cells. An imbalance that leads to an increase in the bad bacteria in the gut can confuse the immune system, causing it to start attacking our own cells, making it a sure-fire route to sickness.

## The Final Word

The focus, thus, should be to score and maintain gut balance tilted towards the good bacteria. People who lead long, healthy and robust lives usually have a very varied, diverse and healthy microbiota.

**Good to Know**
Those who suffer from inflammatory
conditions and lead sickly lives, tend to have
a less diverse microbiome. So they need
to be even more careful.

---

### TO-DO

- Eat healthy consistently. This is important not just to score enough nutrients but also because when we don't eat healthy over a period of time, this could change the composition of our gut microbiome and negatively affect the gut. This mess up leads to inadequate absorption of the nutrients that we need from the food we eat.

- Eat the right foods. This is important because if you eat only junk food (such as pizzas, burgers, doughnuts, etc.) or foods high in unhealthy fats, then the bacteria that help digest these foods will thrive, and others, for example, those that are needed to digest fruit will lose out. Thus, the unhealthy bacteria will outnumber the good bacteria and completely skew the delicate balance in our gut.

- Avoid foods that harm the gut. There are foods that are good for the gut, and then there are many that can harm the fragile gut bacteria. Avoid processed foods as they contain additives like artificial sweeteners, salt and saturated fats that can lead to severe digestive issues and spoil our gut health.

- Eat a wide variety of foods. There are different kinds of bacteria to digest different kinds of foods; the ones that help digest vegetables are different from the ones that work on meats. If you eat only one kind of food, the other bacteria go into hibernation and eventually die out. Eating different kinds of foods not only helps your body absorb the many micronutrients but also ensures diversity of bacteria in your gut. A diverse microbiome is good for you, so ensure that you eat a variety of foods.

- Eat more fibre. Dietary fibre from foods like fruits, grains, nuts and vegetables is the best fuel for maintaining the population of good bacteria in the gut. They help to regulate the digestive tract, promote regular bowel movements and support the good bacteria in the gut.

- When you don't eat fibre-rich foods, the number of bacteria that digest the fibre in the gut decreases, thus impacting the diversity of the gut bacteria negatively. When the bacteria digest the fibre, they produce short-chain fatty acids that nourish the gut, improve immunity and prevent inflammation.

- The connection is simple—more fibre in your diet leads to more fibre-digesting bacteria colonizing the gut. So, a fibre rich diet is a win-win. This also means it is important to avoid processed foods that are often completely devoid of fibre.

- Cook your food right. Minimally processed foods are better for the gut. Therefore lightly sautéed, steamed and raw foods are better for the gut bacteria than fried and overcooked dishes.

- Choose good fats. The types of fats you eat can drastically change the kind of bacteria that decide to live in the intestines. A diet that focuses on good fats, monounsaturated fatty acids (MUFAs) and omega-3 fatty acid helps create a healthier gut.

- Focus on probiotics. Probiotics act as a booster to our digestive health. These are healthy bacteria that work to break down fibre in the body and help rectify the good versus bad bacteria balance in our gut. A diet rich in prebiotic fruits, pulses and vegetables helps to strengthen the probiotics in the gut to further boost our immunity.

- Stay hydrated. Not drinking enough water can dehydrate your gut and lead to chronic constipation which can mess up the gut, and be detrimental to the immunity. So it's important to drink plenty of fluids throughout the day. In fact, those who suffer from constipation, acidity or any other gut malfunction need to be especially careful about their water intake because, along with their gut, their immunity is bound to be at risk as well.

- Avoid these. Alcohol can disrupt the balance of good

and bad bacteria in our gut. It may also increase the production of acid in your stomach, leading to heartburn and acid reflux. Caffeine can also disrupt the balance of good and bad bacteria in the gut; however, if taken in moderation (only 1–2 cups per day), there is no harm.

- Practise stress management. Techniques like practising mindfulness, breathing exercises, carving out some me-time to centre oneself mentally and physically, all help the gut function better.
- Physical activity helps. Exercise helps to move food through the digestive tract. So, engaging in 30 minutes of physical activity, at least, five times a week can promote a healthy gut biome, lead to regular bowel movements and help reduce inflammation in the gut.
- Sleep is just as important. Believe it or not, but our gut bacteria have a circadian rhythm as well. So when we don't sleep, the bugs inside our gut don't sleep. And they too, like us, need sleep to stay efficient. So, have sufficient sleep for the sake of your gut bacteria.

**Fun Fact:** We would fart more if we didn't have good bacteria in our gut!

# 9

# Do Oil Pulling

I spend around 10 minutes every day without fail on my morning ritual of coconut oil pulling. I learnt this practice during my stay at an ayurvedic spa and felt so good that I never stopped. I had read about it and heard about it from many people earlier, but had not been tempted to try it out till then. The proof of the pudding, as they say, is in its taste, after all.

## Why Do You Need to Do Oil Pulling?

The idea of swishing a mouthful of oil around for good oral hygiene might sound strange, but this simple practice called oil pulling is not just a fantastic oral detoxification procedure that makes our teeth whiter, but can actually improve our overall health too. The reason for this is simple—the health of our mouth is in sync with the rest of our body, so when we keep our mouth clean and healthy, the rest of the body follows the lead.

Oil pulling, done typically with coconut oil, sunflower oil or sesame oil, has ancient origins. (The choice of oil is very individual. All of them work equally well.) Pulling is mentioned prominently in the Ayurveda texts, but it is only in the recent times that it has resurfaced, gaining worldwide acceptance as a well-being practice.

Besides the fact that after oil pulling your teeth will feel polished throughout the day as if you have just come from the dentist, this also leads to improved oral hygiene, cavity prevention, removal of toxins from oral cavity and prevention of plaque adherence on the teeth. Daily oil pulling helps fight harmful bacterial and fungal infection, cut inflammation, leads to stronger gums, tongue, teeth, jaw and facial muscles, and heals and prevents bleeding gums. And there's more! It also treats bad breath, relieves dry throat and prevents cracked lips.

## The Modus Operandi

Toxins and bacteria build-up in our mouth over time and cause dental plaque if they are not removed regularly. Oil pulling literally helps 'pull' them out of our mouth. Oil actually helps to bind, trap and eliminate the microorganisms from the deep pockets within the teeth and gums and the difficult to reach regions around root canals.

**Good to Know**

Bad bacteria build-up in our mouth can actually up our risk for heart disease, so this practice is said to be good for our heart too.

## The Immunity Connection

Oil pulling helps boost our immune system too. According to Ayurveda, oil pulling is said to cure multiple systemic diseases (ones that can affect the entire body, for example, flu, high blood pressure, infections etc.) when practised regularly.

It helps to purify the entire system as according to Ayurvedic medicine, each section of the tongue is connected to different organs such as kidneys, lungs, liver, heart, small intestines, stomach, colon and spine.

It also helps reduce inflammation in the gums and oral tissues and detoxify the body, and have a direct positive connection with our immunity.

Western medicine does not recognize the merits of this ancient practice and research proving these claims are few. However, the benefits are clear for everyone to see. Also, there is no harm done and there are no apparent side effects, so this natural method is definitely worth a try.

---

### TO-DO

- There are two ways to practise oil pulling. The first one, Gandusha, involves filling the mouth completely with oil, holding it in for about three to five minutes and then spitting it out. The more popular method, Kavalgraha, involves holding the little quantity of oil in the mouth and swishing and gargling for anywhere between five to 20 minutes, then spitting it out quickly.
- Oil pulling should be done first thing in the morning, ideally every day before eating or drinking anything.
- It is important to not swallow the oil during or after the practice as during the process it takes all the bacteria and toxins from the mouth which should not enter the system again.
- After spitting, one can rinse the mouth with water and brush as usual. To take the process up a notch, after oil pulling, scrape the tongue with a good tongue scraper to get that bacteria-laden gunk right off to supercharge your immunity.

**Fun Fact:** Oil pulling originated in India as part of natural healing practices described in ancient Ayurveda texts (one was written in 800 BC and the other in 700 BC).

# IMMUNITY DOWNERS

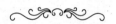

# 10

# Watch Your Weight

I have spent more than 25 years working in a private nutrition practice. I have worked with some really smart women and men—people who are running huge, successful businesses, people who other people look up to, celebrities in different fields, including acting and modelling. All of them are people who seem like they can do anything they want.

And yet they don't. When it comes to their health and weight, they too, often fail like most of us do. Many of them suffer from issues like overeating, binge eating, emotional eating and more. They often have poor body images and are riddled with self-doubt and are forever upset about what they eat and how they look.

So the fact is that no matter how successful or famous or moneyed we are, so many of us are hungry for real answers when it comes to nutrition and eating right. And an even bigger problem is that our heads are filled with unachievable standards of how a 'perfect' body should look. That is why most people keep looking for the perfect solution—a perfect body! The truth is that there is no 'one' perfect body that'll fit all! But there is an optimum weight that everyone can aspire for and work towards.

## Why Do You Need to Watch Your Weight?

Is it because you want to look good when you go to a beach holiday? Or a college reunion is coming up and you don't want to look wasted? Or has your family history of diabetes or high cholesterol or your aching knees finally alarmed you?

There are as many reasons as there are people who want to shed weight. But one very important reason to want to get to the optimum weight is missed by almost every one—better immunity.

Most of us know that obesity negatively impacts our blood sugar, cholesterol and blood pressure, and can also play a role in increasing cancer, sleep apnea, fatty liver disease among other disorders. However, the connection of excess weight with immunity is far less discussed.

## The Immunity Connection

Obesity actually is an extremely complex phenomenon (disorder) that alters multiple processes and pathways in the body, any of which could affect and sabotage our immune system. This, of course, is a study in progress, but some effects are understood well already. Every extra kilogram you carry translates to one extra kilogram of tissue that the immune cells must defend and take care of—which is why being overweight is linked to reduced immune activity.

Overweight people have lowered levels of lymphocytes (infection-fighting WBCs), more killer cell dysfunction and decreased cytokine production, all of which are imperative for the efficient functioning of the system. Excess body fat can actually inhibit the ability of WBCs to multiply, produce antibodies and prevent inflammation.

Obesity leads to low-grade, chronic inflammation in body fat tissue and keeps the immune system in a permanently switched-on mode. Higher levels of the white adipose tissue (WAT)—the type of fat that shows up as unwanted bulges around our thighs, arms and belly—in the body lead to an increased production of inflammatory cytokines, keeping our body's immune system permanently switched on. This compromises the immune system's efficiency and makes it harder for the body to fight off the infections when they actually occur.

### Good to Know

Anyone can be at risk, depending on their body fat percentage, not their weight. It is possible to have a 'normal' BMI (and be of normal weight) and still have a lot of excess fat (called skinny fat). The skinny-fat people are at risk for inflammation and a faulty immune system too.

Finally, very often obese people tend to be deficient in important immunity boosting nutrients because of a poor diet. Deficiencies can occur in anyone who eats poorly, no matter their weight, but the chances of missing detection is higher in people who are overweight because of the wrong social perception—fat people are eating enough and hence cannot face deficiencies.

The good news though is that when overweight people lose weight, their lymphocyte levels and function improve dramatically.

- Instead of trying to get skinny, focus on gaining a healthy body composition. Work on two main areas: sufficiently developed muscle mass and a body fat percentage in a healthy range, which is 10–20 per cent for men and 18–28 per cent for women.
- Watch out for yo-yo dieting (repeatedly losing, then regaining weight) because it stresses the body and prevents the immunity cells from defending the body against invading bacteria or viruses and can have a lasting negative impact on the immunity.
- Work towards achieving your target weight and then maintain it there.

**Fun Fact:** Obesity is linked to more than 60 chronic diseases.

# 11

# Don't Self-Medicate

Have you felt a blocked nose coming on and gulped down a medicine for cold on the advice of your local chemist, basing your decision on hearsay or trusting some advertisement? Do you pop painkillers all the time, without a second thought? If your answer is 'yes' to both, then you, like many others, are self-medicating.

Isn't everyone, almost everyone you know, right from your office colleagues to your neighbour, a self-proclaimed medical authority? Just utter the words 'fever', 'cold', 'cough', 'constipation' or 'indigestion', and your friends or even total strangers will provide unsolicited advice on which medicines work best and which are useless. It's highly probable that you too have a ready repertoire of remedies.

Self-medication can be defined in simple terms, as the use of medicines by a person to treat a perceived or real health problem without consulting a physician. Medicines for self-medication are often called 'non-prescription' or 'over the counter' (OTC) medicines and are available without a doctor's prescription in most pharmacies.

The most common reasons for choosing to self-medicate are:

- Lack of time for an appointment with a physician
- Increase in the cost of healthcare

- A relative or friend's advice to buy a particular medicine based on their experience
- Increased awareness about different types of medicines
- Tendency to look for fast symptomatic relief

There is no doubt that we are overmedicated. There are just too many OTC medicines available and many people consider self-treatment with OTC medicines an easy, cheaper and hassle-free alternative to visiting the doctor. Any temporary relief they find only reinforces this habit. So, the dangers of self-medication are ignored blatantly.

## Why Do We Need to Stop Self-Medication?

Self-diagnosis and self-medication can only go so far and can have serious repercussions on our health. The seemingly innocuous drugs that we take often have several side effects that are asymptomatic, but might lead to some internal disorder. For example, painkillers and cold remedies may cause acidity, fluid retention, increase in blood pressure, and even kidney damage. In fact, arbitrary intake of anti-inflammatory painkillers can prove to be fatal. These medicines may cause the platelet count to drop so low that the chances of fatality can skyrocket.

Allergy to drugs is another red flag. Often people do not read the label properly before taking medicines; a typical case in point are cough syrups and they can cause various allergies.

It is also possible to become addicted to OTCs—when people stop taking them abruptly, severe withdrawal symptoms can occur. It is also important to know about the medicine's possible side effects and the food, drinks and other medicines to avoid while popping a pill.

## Good to Know

Self-medication often delays proper treatment of the disease. It may give temporary, superficial relief and in the process, mask the symptoms, possibly indicative of a more serious problem.

## The Immunity Connection

Self-medication undermines the immune system too. Bacteria in the body continue to do what they do best—adapt in order to survive so they tend to outsmart the ingested antibiotics and have the amazing and scary ability to even mutate to build defences against the drugs. Do this too often and this may lead to an increasing incidence of antimicrobial resistance (AMR).

Simply put, each time you take a round of antibiotics, especially when you don't need it, it boosts the spread of resistance by giving harmful bugs the opportunity to adapt to the drugs. Besides, antibiotics, in addition to the bad bacteria, also end up killing the good bacteria in the body, which messes up the good vs bad bacteria balance in the gut and is a sure-fire way to lower the immunity, making it difficult to fight off further infections.

## TO-DO

- Practise responsible self-medication. Try not to self-medicate all the time and only take the medicines after being well-informed about their safe and effective use in response to a particular condition.
- It is important to realize that just because medicines are available over the counter, it does not mean that they are risk-free. Also, just a label that says 'organic' or 'natural'

in big green letters is not a sign that the medication is safe. You can have an adverse reaction to anything, even supplements.

- It is necessary to consult a doctor each time you suspect an infection, rather than taking antibiotics on whim, following an earlier prescription or using leftover medicines. Always remember that similar symptoms in different people may require different medicines and only your doctor can decide which course of antibiotics is suitable for you.
- Use antibiotics only when necessary—that is, to treat serious, confirmed bacterial infections and life-threatening diseases. Your doctor is trained to take that call for you.
- The next time you reach out for an antihistamine, a sleeping pill, a painkiller or an antibiotic without consulting a doctor, be mindful of the side effects.

**Fun Fact:** In the year 1945, Sir Alexander Fleming, who had discovered penicillin in 1928, warned the world that overusing antibiotics, particularly at low doses, could lead to widespread resistance.

## 12

# Keep Inflammation Down

Inflammation sounds like a really loaded word, difficult to understand and fathom. Most of all, it is confusing—is it good for us or bad? Does it help or harm our internal systems?

Let me try and explain in simple terms. The red bump on your skin that is a result of a mosquito bite or a bee sting is a sign of inflammation in your body. Pain, swelling, warm feeling on the skin, often, even loss of function—these are all signs of an acute infection which is usually temporary and lasts for a few hours to a few days. These symptoms occur when the body responds by increasing blood flow to the damaged area and releases chemicals, antibodies and proteins. As soon as the healing occurs, the symptoms disappear.

Then there is chronic inflammation, which typically refers to inflammation that lasts longer than six months. The damage or infection is ongoing, causing continuous inflammation that can slowly injure blood vessels, nerves and organs (like the kidney), as well as joints, skin and even the brain.

The scary part about chronic inflammation is that you may not feel any pain because many organs do not have pain receptors, but the inflammation may turn out to be life threatening.

## Why Do We Need to Keep Inflammation Down?

When the immune response is constantly and repeatedly triggered, and our bodies are constantly inflamed, this leads to cumulative damage that often adds up to diseases like Type 2 diabetes, heart disease, Alzheimer's, cancer and depression. Other disorders like arthritis, liver disease, osteoporosis, cancer, asthma, allergies, irritable bowel syndrome and early ageing can also be traced to high levels of inflammation in our body.

The crux of the matter is that when long-term, chronic inflammation settles in the body, it is likely to be detrimental to our health. So, the idea is to keep a check on chronic inflammation to ensure that we don't fall seriously sick.

## The Immunity Connection

Inflammation plays a vital role in our body. It makes our immune system active and leads to quick redressal of everyday bruises and abrasions. Without inflammation, we would succumb to infections, surgeries and injuries, and get diseases more frequently. Simply put, without inflammation, we would not survive.

**Good to Know**

Inflammation, thus, is part of our immune system's defence mechanism and plays an essential role in healing and keeping infections at bay.

---

### TO-DO

You can effectively put a lid on inflammation by following some simple food rules.

- Inflammation is usually fuelled by our overly acidic bodies, thanks to our wrong eating habits (we consume many acidic foods like caffeine, alcohol, processed foods, sugars, refined flours and excess animal products), pollution and stress. We must ensure that we limit our consumption of these foods.
- Keep the body alkaline by eating an alkalizing diet, i.e., consume more vegetables and fruits.
- Eat lots of fibre as it cuts inflammation by helping lower C-reactive protein (CRP) levels in the blood, and by feeding good bacteria to the gut. Focus on fruits, vegetables and whole grains.
- Avoid junk and processed foods as most of these are loaded with high-fructose corn syrup, trans fats and have too much sodium, all festering inflammation in the body.
- Cut down on added sugar consciously. It severely suppresses the immune system, making us vulnerable to inflammatory disorders. High fructose diets and sugar diets are known to damage mitochondria and shift the liver from burning fat to storing it, besides increasing the inflammation. Avoid refined sugars, aerated drinks and artificial sweeteners. Also, you can even try opting for natural sugars like jaggery and honey.
- Spice up. Add anti-inflammatory herbs and spices like turmeric, ginger and cinnamon to your diet liberally to boost antioxidants intake; they help tame inflammation.
- Eat good fats. Correct the omega-3 and omega-6 fatty acids ratio. Omega-3 suppresses inflammatory chemicals in the body, whereas too much omega-6 does the opposite. You can get omega-3 in your diet through fatty fish such as salmon and mackerel, flaxseeds and walnuts. To bring omega-6 down, eat less meat and reduce the consumption of refined oil.

- Drink green tea. It is rich in a compound called epigallocatechin gallate (EGCG) that helps cut down inflammation by reducing production of the pro-inflammatory compound, cytokine, in the body.
- Treat acute inflammation by managing it, not trying to cure it. For the first 24–48 hours, follow the RICE method: rest, ice, compression and elevation. Take limited doses of a painkiller like ibuprofen recommended by your doctor. Rest and give your body time to heal. Too many painkillers and other anti-inflammatory medications may actually prevent recovery and may lead to persistent pain and instability.
- Here are five simple tips to follow everyday:
  - Include vegetables in every meal. Snack on two fruits a day and eat at least three servings of raw foods every day.
  - Eat a variety of foods. Try to include as many colours of the rainbow in your diet. A simple rule of thumb—more colours mean more antioxidants.
  - Restrict intake of processed and junk foods to once a week.
  - Snack on nuts and seeds every day.
  - Get adequate sleep—both quality and duration of sleep directly impact inflammation.

**Fun Fact:** Don't skip meals as too many peaks and drops in blood sugar may lead to inflammation in the body.

13

# Beat the Pollution

If you live in a metropolitan city, you're already familiar with the headlines regarding air quality: 'Hold your breath, today's air quality could be the season's worst'. You read these in the papers early in the morning with your morning cup of tea and then go on to digest lists of primary pollutants in the air, statistics about how the pollution is at an all-time high, and pore over the adverse effects of breathing in unhealthy amounts of particulate matter.

## Why Do We Need to Beat the Pollution?

Everyday we rue the fact that we are helpless about the situation and go out and breathe in the same air we have been warned about every single day. The assault, by the way is equally bad indoors.

Meanwhile our stress levels are skyrocketing, reading the air quality index (AQI) every day, our lungs bear the maximum brunt when it comes to poor air quality because that's where the toxic matter we breathe in gets lodged. Some of us show adverse reactions to polluted air even with short-term exposure, and in the long run, it can cause respiratory and cardiac distress. But that's not all! Our immunity takes a huge hit as well.

## The Immunity Connection

Inhaling dirty air loaded with tiny pollution particles can trigger the release of WBCs into the bloodstream and lead to inflammation—a sure-fire immunity downer (see the chapter on inflammation).

Some of the substances we inhale have the ability to change the natural composition of gut microbes, tipping the balance towards the harmful ones. And as we've discussed already, when the precarious balance of microbes tilts in favour of the harmful bacteria, it can lead to an errant immune response (see the chapter on gut health).

**Good to Know**
Our immunological development and maturation starts even when we are a developing foetus, during our mothers pregnancy. Exposure of the mother to pollution at this critical stage can modify immune responses and cells, and influence the risk of allergies and other immune diseases in the unborn child too.

So what concrete action can we take to combat the environmental toxicity besides complaining, whining about it, writing lengthy posts on social media, blaming everybody. We cannot just run away and move to a remote corner of the world, can we? That's not an option for most of us.

What we *can* do is work on strengthening our lungs and reducing our exposure, and thus, the harm caused, so that we can face these polluted times better. The answer lies in identifying and tackling the culprits.

- Set a healthy weight target and work towards it consistently. Overweight people breathe more air per day than those with a healthy weight, which makes them more vulnerable to air contaminants and respiratory irritants such as ammonia, sulfur dioxide, ozone and nitrogen dioxide. Get your weight in check to minimize the damage of pollution on yourself.

- Cut the smoke. Our bodies do not like cigarette smoke; it causes damage, disease and cuts days off your life. Quitting smoking is by far the most important thing you can do to keep your lungs healthy in these toxic times when breathing the air itself is equivalent to smoking several cigarettes a day. Here's why:

  o The inside of our lungs is lined with tiny, hair-like structures called cilia which push the debris and microbes out of our lungs to keep us safe. When smoke enters the lungs and respiratory tract, it paralyses the cilia, which leads to the toxins accumulating in the lungs. This results in excessive mucus production, causing respiratory infections and lung diseases, and subsequently, messing up our immunity.

  o Passive smoking will damage your lungs as much as smoking. So be strict about avoiding smoke in all forms.

  o If your partner is a smoker, make a pact that they don't smoke around you. In fact, actively try to get them to quit. If you get many visitors who smoke, put stickers forbidding smoking next to the main entrance of the house, the dashboard of the car, living room... everywhere! Your space and life are more important than any offence they might take.

- o Be wary of toxic fumes. Breathe in through your nose, especially around toxic fumes. The hair in your nose acts as a filter and only lets extremely fine particles through, keeping heavier particulate out.
- Try to take shallow breaths so that the fumes don't travel deep into your lungs. Once you're in the clear, cough hard a few times to expel them. Car exhaust and gasoline fumes, tobacco smoke and regular smoke, cleaning supplies, paint, talcum or baby powder (has tiny, crushed rocks that stay on in your lungs) are all toxic to breathe in, so ideally, try to avoid them in the first place.
- Avoid pesticides. Pesticides can enter our bodies through skin contact, ingestion (they can remain on vegetables and fruits), or inhalation. Obviously, if pesticides can kill living organisms, they can harm us too. The best way to avoid air pollution from pesticides is not to use them at all. Instead, use more eco-friendly products and wash fruits and vegetables properly before use.
- Clean air inside our homes is fundamental to good health. Most of us spend a lot of our time indoors, so indoor air pollution can be even deadlier than outdoor air pollution. Poor indoor air quality can exacerbate allergies and asthma, cause eye, nose and throat irritation, or lead to fatigue, nausea or illness. All this can result in not just poor work performance and productivity but may also undermine your well-being and, of course, your immunity.
- Here are a few simple steps that can help:
- o Adopt the tradition from generations past and leave your shoes at the door. Not only is going barefoot very comfortable, but you also reduce the dirt you bring into the house. Alternatively, keep indoor slippers

separate from outdoor footwear.

- ○ Improve your home's indoor air quality by opening the windows frequently for some cross ventilation. Install exhaust vents in the kitchen and all bathrooms.
- ○ Consider getting air-purifying plants for your home. Boston Fern, Areca Palm, English Ivy, Peace Lily, Australian Sword Fern and Rubber Plants can all thrive indoors and help lower indoor air pollution.

- Soak in the greens. Living in crowded areas is actually a double whammy. It makes us prone to contracting crowd infections (viral infections), which cause more inflammation and thus leads to the possibility of inflammatory diseases like asthma and irritable bowel syndrome. Meanwhile, it also prevents us from scoring the beneficial impact that exposure to environmental microbes, like those found in rural environments, farms and green spaces, has on strengthening our immune systems.

  Exposure to these friendly microbes plays a vital role in guarding against inflammatory disorders. That is why people living in urban areas with less access to green spaces are more likely to have chronic inflammation, which is caused by immune system dysfunction. So, the solution for city dwellers is to avoid crowd infections by not only taking care of their hygiene, but also finding ways to increase their exposure to 'old friends' by visiting green spaces that would allow their immune systems to come into contact with more beneficial microbes.

  It is easier said than done, but a fine balance needs to be maintained. In fact, exposure to the farm environment in childhood, and even prenatally, has been shown to decrease the risk of allergic diseases in people.

- Turn to yoga. One of the best things you can do for your

lungs is to strike a yoga pose. It'll help offset the pollution damage. Kapalbhati Kriya and Bhastrika Pranayam help remove all the toxins stuck in the nasal tract and lungs and throw them out forcefully in the form of cough. Utthita Hasta Padasana is another important yoga pose. Stand with your feet spread three to four feet apart. Then extend your hands to the sides from the shoulders towards the wrist and knuckles. It helps open out the ribcage, expands the chest muscles and enhances breathing.

- Get moving! Regular physical exercise is good for your whole body and especially, your lungs. It makes the muscles around your lungs work harder and makes them stronger. You will find a difference within a couple of weeks of doing cardio.
- Junk the junk and get fruit power. It's not just the air you breathe, what you eat has a lot to do with saving yourself from pollution too. Here are a few simple foods to try:
  - Get apple power for your lungs. Apples help improve the lung capacity and reduce wheezing, thanks to the flavonoids quercetin and khellin, which help open up stuffed airways.
  - Load up on vitamin C. This vitamin helps arrest the damage caused to lung tissue by environmental toxins. So make sure you have an amla (Indian gooseberry) or two oranges daily.
  - Score some resveratrol. Now, if grapes are not in season, you can get it from peanuts. It helps cut the inflammation and keep the lungs fighting.
  - Low potassium levels are linked to shortness of breath, so zero in on high potassium foods like banana and other fruits.
  - Pineapple is a good bet too. The enzyme bromelain in

it helps clear out the toxic debris that accumulates in the lungs and thus helps it detox naturally.

- o Ginger is a proven remedy (begin your day with a cup of ginger tea and have another when you get back home after work); it helps stamp air pollutants out of the air passages before they get the time to irritate the lungs.

- o Add mint to your fresh juice and sprinkle oregano in your breakfast omelette (or besan cheela, stir fries). They have antihistamines that work as antidotes for symptoms like nasal congestion, mucous formation and sneezing.

- o Finally, always keep a clove under your tongue (and keep sucking on it slowly) when you step out. An organic expectorant, clove helps to break up phlegm in the throat and esophagus, and also helps prevent respiratory tract infections. Drinking clove tea too is a great idea.

**Fun Fact:** Being shut inside a car may not protect you from pollution. In fact, you can be exposed to more bad air than a cyclist. When driving in heavy traffic, use the recycled-air setting on your fan so that the car does not suck in toxic fumes.

# III

## EAT THE RIGHT FOODS

14

# Focus on Fibre

Till now, you may have been asked to increase your fibre intake for reasons varying from keeping constipation away to keeping your heart healthy, besides adding a tasty crunch to the food you eat. Now there's another motivation; if you want profound, positive changes in your immune system, load up on soluble fibre.

## The Effects

Fibre is the most underrated ingredient around; in fact, most people consider it just a bulk-adding part of our meals, whereas the truth is that fibre is our best friend. We just can't ignore it.

That's because fibre equals satiety. It keeps our stomach full for long on lesser calories and helps keep hunger in check. It also slows digestion by forming a gel-like combination along with water in the stomach, which slackens the rate at which foods are emptied from the abdomen.

Also, when you slow down digestion, you slow the delivery of glucose (blood sugar) to the bloodstream, leading to less insulin being released, which helps lower the fat-storage rate, particularly in the belly (which directly translates to slimmer waists). It is essential here to understand that insulin spike tells our body to start storing fat, and the spike is invariably followed by a drop that leaves us feeling tired and hungry and wanting to eat more. Fibre in the diet helps avoid this vicious cycle.

## The Immunity Connection

Fibre supports our immunity by supporting digestion, encouraging regular bowel movement and boosting the production of good bacteria in the gut.

Bacteria in our gut break down consumed fibre and produce short-chain fatty acids that help cut inflammation in the body.

Beta-glucan, a form of soluble dietary fibre that is strongly linked to improving cholesterol levels and boosting heart health, can boost the immune system and protect against free radical damage to our cells, tissues and organs. It also works as an immune modulator i.e. it 'modulates' or 'changes' the immune system to make it as efficient as possible by alerting immune system cells in the body to destroy foreign microorganisms.

Soluble fibre leads to increased production of an anti-inflammatory protein called interleukin-4 which helps us recover faster from infection. So, whether or not you are eating oats, apples, nuts, seeds, strawberries, carrots, citrus fruits and barley—all good sources of soluble fibre—can determine how well you will be able to fight against the rampant diseases and also how soon you'll recover.

**Good to Know**

Soluble fibre also changes the personality of immune cells—they go from being pro-inflammatory, angry cells to anti-inflammatory, healing cells that help us recover faster from infection.

It is important to understand that while insoluble fibre (found in whole wheat and whole-grain products, wheat bran and green, leafy vegetables) is of great value for the body as it provides bulk and satiety to give a boost to the immune system, we need to load up consciously on soluble fibre.

## TO-DO

- Eating fruit and vegetables are the easiest and most practical way of getting fibre. You must fix your eating window. For example, an apple after breakfast, a plateful of papaya in the evening or a couple of oranges and a plateful of sautéed vegetables with dinner will ensure that you get enough fibre easily.
- The wider the variety of plant fibre you eat, the healthier and 'more diverse' the bacteria in the gut will be. The optimum level of variety is eating 30 different types of fruit and vegetables per week, including nuts, seeds and herbs. It is not as difficult to follow as it sounds.
- Another excellent trick is to grind flaxseeds, sunflower, sesame or pumpkin seeds and almonds to a fine powder, and eat two tablespoons of this powder daily. You can even routinely add seeds to your cereal, soups, yoghurt to feel fuller.
- Incorporate lentils, whole grain cereals (brown rice, whole bread, oats, barley, etc.) and beans consciously in your diet.
- One important piece of advice I'd like to give here is to eat some fibre in the mornings during breakfast as that helps avoid the hunger pangs in the afternoon. However, make sure you drink enough fluids throughout the day to ensure that fibre works efficiently in the body.

**Fun Fact:** Unlike fat, protein and carbohydrates, fibre has almost nil calories.

15

# The Spicy Truth

India is known as the 'home of spices'. There is no other country that produces as many kinds of spices as India. There are over 80 different spices grown in different parts of the world and around 50 spices are grown in India. Though many nations love hot sauces and hot foods, spices and India go a long way back. And today, too, the 'spice-box' is an intrinsic part of an Indian kitchen.

But spices don't just exist to make our food palatable. When used in the right way, they can be just the tool that can pave the way towards a disease preventive plan, creating an iron-clad immunity that can shield us from infections and myriad bacteria and viruses. The best news is that every spice has something good going for it. So, it's time to stock up your spice rack.

## The Effects

Spices add the necessary micronutrients to the diet. They supply disease-fighting antioxidants in bulk. They also help you eat more of the foods you don't otherwise like and thus help reap their benefits.

# The Immunity Connection

Not only do spices add zing to what you eat but they are also potent immune system warriors. Ayurveda, the ancient system of healing, has used spices as remedies for their curative properties for centuries now. And today, spices can be our saviour in these turbulent times and build up our immunity against various viruses that have been recently cropping up. While almost all spices help boost immunity, some help more than others.

## Turmeric

Turmeric has curcumin, an antiviral and a strong fighter against cold and flu. Curcumin also helps lower the levels of inflammatory enzymes (caused due to infection) in your body and is incredibly purifying. Loaded with antioxidants, tumeric is antifungal, antimicrobial, antibacterial and helps keep infection at bay.

## Cumin Seeds

Cumin seeds are a good source of iron, a mineral that is an integral component of haemoglobin and transports oxygen from the lungs to all body cells; it is important for energy production and metabolism. Additionally, iron also helps keep the immune system healthy.

## Black Pepper

Black pepper is both an antioxidant and an antibacterial agent and thus contributes to overall wellness tremendously. It also has vitamin C, which naturally boosts immunity, and works as an excellent antibiotic.

## Clove

An organic expectorant, clove helps break up phlegm in the throat and oesophagus. It also helps prevent respiratory tract infections.

## Carom Seeds

Carom seeds help in treating cold and warding off nasal blockage and flu. They also help effectively deal with respiratory ailments associated with various types of flu. They are high in thymol, which increases the secretion of gastric juices and helps us absorb food, thus the immunity-boosting nutrients better.

## Sun-Dried Fenugreek Leaves

This lesser-known spice doesn't just add an amazing umami flavour to dishes, but is also an excellent source of fibre. Fenugreek leaves are known to be an effective cholesterol and inflammation cutter in the body. They also keep digestion running smoothly which is essential for good immunity and keeping blood sugar in check.

## Coriander Powder

Coriander powder is excellent for relieving flatulence and aiding better digestion by facilitating smoother bowel movement and that is why it has been used extensively in our traditional dishes since ancient times. Good gut health ensures not only protection against the cold virus but faster recovery from an infection.

## Garam Masala

This is a blend of ground whole spices and is full of antioxidants that help boost digestion and fight inflammation in the body, thus keeping our immunity at its optimum. It is also full of antioxidants and fights bloating and flatulence.

*Tip: Make sure you source garam masala that has all these spices in it: fennel, bay leaves, black and white peppercorns, cloves, cinnamon, mace, black and green cardamom pods, cumin, coriander seeds, and red chilli powder.*

### Saffron

This spice helps in the proliferation of T-cells and elevates the level of the antioxidant glutathione in the blood, which affects immunity positively.

**Good to Know**

Spices are a very cost-effective, culturally acceptable and sustainable way of eating well and staying healthy. Just a tiny pinch goes a long way.

---

TO-DO

Get adventurous with spices and cook up a storm of flavours! The best news is that spices can be added to any recipe and any food, be it soups, breads, mustards, marinades, butters, sauces, salad dressings, stocks, vinegars, desserts or drinks.

- Warm up some milk, add some powdered turmeric to it and a pinch of pepper and drink it at night before going to sleep. If milk does not work for you, just add some turmeric to warm water with ginger and pepper (both potent infection busters) and begin your day fighting fit.
- Make energy booster bars by combining turmeric, ghee, pepper and jaggery. Eat one every day.
- Eat 2 grams of pan-roasted carom seeds every day. Or

have carom tea: boil water, add black or green tea, add carom seeds, ginger and cardamom. Add milk and let the mixture boil well for about 3 minutes.

- Add clove to your tea or the glass of warm milk you drink at night before bed.

**Fun Fact:** Saffron is one of the most expensive spices in the world. This is because the vibrant, thread-like spice is harvested by hand.

# 16

# Hydrate Enough

Have you ever felt tired and listless for no reason? Do you wonder why you cannot lose weight even after diet restrictions and enough exercise? And why you fall sick so often? Well, the answers may be more obvious than you think.

Your water intake can affect how your body functions. Here's my secret: I make a water plan for every client and help them steadily build up to optimum drinking measures in a few weeks. When they reach the optimum level, without fail, their reaction is: 'I am feeling so much better, have so much more energy. I don't know why I was not drinking enough water earlier!'

Water is the cornerstone of life, as every cell of the human body is dependent on it. It regulates body temperature, removes waste, helps carry nutrients and oxygen to cells, converts food to energy, facilitates the absorption of nutrients from the food we eat, protects and cushions vital organs, and moistens oxygen for breathing.

Yet, we forget to drink enough water in the rush of our day. Also, most people don't really understand the importance of staying hydrated and pay a big price for this folly. This is precisely why water is called the 'forgotten nutrient'.

## The Effects

Lack of water is the number one trigger of daytime fatigue. Our muscles need a proper electrolyte-water balance in the body, so even mild dehydration can slow down our efficiency. The quickest way, in fact, to increase energy is to consume water!

Drinking enough water may be the most crucial piece to the weight-loss puzzle. That is because adequate water ensures that both our digestion and metabolism work at full capacity, which is essential to ensure weight maintenance (or loss).

Dehydration may also lead to brain fog, make your internal systems and organs sluggish, cause myriad health issues like kidney stones and down your immunity too—a connection most people do not know about.

## The Immunity Connection

Dehydration is a common immunity downer for multiple reasons. First, drinking water helps improve cognitive function, leading to healthier and safer everyday decisions, a prerequisite to leading a healthy lifestyle.

Second, drinking enough water ensures that the mucous membranes in our mouth and nose stay moist. Moisture prevents dust, viruses and bacteria from sticking to tissue and from entering our body and causing harm. Mucous is our body's first line of defence against intruders, so to ensure your mucus membranes are adequately hydrated, drink lots of water.

Third, sweating is one of the main ways our bodies remove contaminants (toxins, waste, bacteria) from circulation in the body before they have a chance to become a full-blown infection.

Fourth, being well hydrated is essential for the functioning of the lymphatic system, which works closely with our immune system. A well-functioning lymphatic system helps remove toxins, waste, debris, abnormal cells and pathogens from the body. It also helps to transport infection-fighting WBCs throughout the body. Lower body water content may mean less lymph production as this clear and colourless fluid comprises about 90 per cent water.

Fifth, the more water we drink, the better our kidneys operate in flushing out any unwelcome toxins through urination. Smoothly functioning kidneys ensure that our immune system is not weakened or weighed down by the unnecessary toxins residing in the body.

Sixth, water lubricates the digestive organs and assists in breaking down foods and increasing nutrient absorption, which is necessary for a robust immunity system. Our bodies also need water to make stomach acid hydrochloric acid (HCl), whose lesser-known function (besides better digestion) is to eliminate bacteria and viruses in the stomach.

Seventh, our immune system is highly dependent on the nutrients in our bloodstream and our bloodstream is made mostly of water! Not hydrating well hinders the nutrients from getting transported to all organs.

Eighth, drinking plenty of water ensures that our cells get

adequate nutrition from the blood. Water helps to oxygenate the blood in our body, and healthy, happy cells packed with oxygen translate into more efficient working muscles and organs, ensuring superior immunity.

## How Much Water Should You Drink Each Day?

This is a simple question with no easy answer. How much water one should consume varies for each person and also depends on various factors—your health, how active you are, where you live, etc. But on an average, everyone should aim to drink two to three litres of water every day. Another way to ensure your body gets enough water is to drink a minimum of half your body weight in ounces of water; this means if you weigh 120 pounds (54 kilograms), you need to drink about 60 ounces (1.7 litres) of water daily. If you weigh 200 pounds (90 kilograms), you need to drink about 100 ounces (2.9 litres).

**Good to Know**
One must stay hydrated year-round,
not just in the summer months, when we
sweat visibly. Also, you need to drink water
whether you are indoors or outdoors.

Your body needs more water if you

- regularly eat dry, concentrated and fat-rich foods. These foods need more water to ensure digestion.
- regularly eat salty foods. Excess salt in our body is removed through urination.
- are continually stressed. Stress increases metabolism and uses up more water; you might feel thirstier if you are stressed.

- are overweight since basic functions like digestion, blood circulation, etc., will require a larger amount of water.
- regularly consume caffeine and alcohol. Both these drinks are diuretic and can severely dehydrate the body.

*Tip: Follow this rule: for each cup of coffee you take, drink an additional cup of water. For each glass of an alcoholic beverage, drink additional two cups of water.*

## Are You Dehydrated?

The signs and symptoms of dehydration include mild to excessive thirst, fatigue, headache, rapid heartbeat, dry flushed skin, dry mouth, little or no urination, muscle weakness, dizziness, muscle cramps and light-headedness.

*Tip: The best way to tell if you are dehydrated is to check the colour of your urine—if it's dark, you need to drink more, and if it's pale yellow, you are doing fine.*

---

### TO-DO

- Wake up to water—literally. Before you eat or drink anything else in the morning, have a glass or two of water.
- Carry your own bottle of water everywhere you go. Have one in your bag, in your car, etc.
- Don't wait till you're thirsty; keep drinking water regularly throughout the day. Try wearing a digital watch that beeps at the beginning of each hour. Use that as a reminder to pour yourself a glass of water.

- You can follow this simple water plan:
  - Begin your day with two glasses of water.
  - Drink an entire one-litre bottle of water by lunchtime and another by dinnertime.
  - Have a glass of warm water after every meal.
- You can even eat your water. Certain fruits and vegetables, such as cucumbers, celery, leafy vegetables, zucchini, melons, berries and cauliflower are rich in water and can help keep the body adequately hydrated.

Here are some other ways in which you can catch extra hydration throughout the day:

- A veggie-loaded smoothie with breakfast.
- A glass of coconut water as a mid-morning beverage.
- A glass of cool, refreshing buttermilk with lunch.
- Sip on water infused with mint, basil or a citrus fruit throughout the day.
- Water boiled with carom seeds or fennel seeds will hydrate and help boost digestion as well.
- A cup of herbal tea with ginger and pepper in the evening.
- A bowl of soup with dinner.

**Fun Fact:** By the time you feel thirsty, your body has lost more than 1 per cent of its total water. So, keep drinking water regularly.

Kavita Devgan

# 17

# Get the Protein Power

Whyen we talk about critical deficiencies that afflict Indians, along with iron and calcium, protein deficiency tops the list. Unfortunately, most of us don't give protein much thought. The common thinking is that protein is important only for bodybuilders or for people who exercise a lot, whereas the fact is that many of us tend to be deficient in this macronutrient.

When I do a food audit, I am usually told that the staple fare for a vegetarian (often even non vegetarian) person is tomato sandwich or poha for breakfast, dal and chawal for lunch, and roti and two vegetables for dinner. There is very little protein intake in this kind of diet. And what is worse is that nine out of 10 times, people are unaware of the lacuna.

## The Effects

Protein deficiency harms us in more ways than one. Unlike fats and carbohydrates, we need to supply our body with protein daily as it is not stored in the body and its deficiency can thus lead to depletion of our muscle mass. Secondly, every body part is made up of protein, so it is needed for maintenance, upkeep and regeneration of all our body cells and organs—right from hair to hormones, antibodies to nerves and haemoglobin to bones. And, of course, it is needed to keep our immunity strong.

Not many people understand the connection of protein with strengthened immunity. This oversight can mess up immunity for many of us.

## The Immunity Connection

How protein impacts our immunity is clear. It helps form the cells that operate the immune system.

Proteins are made up of hundreds or thousands of smaller units called amino acids, which are interconnected in long chains and are a key factor in the formation of antibodies. As the essential amino acids cannot be synthesized in the body, they must be supplied through our diet and their deficiency affects antibody production negatively.

In addition, an amino acid called cysteine is particularly important as it is involved in the formation of an antioxidant glutathione, which is a potent immunity booster.

So, this is how protein supports a healthy immune system:

- It helps you recover and repair after an illness.
- It helps build antibodies.
- It promotes the synthesis of glutathione.

Another bonus is that many foods high in protein also contain other immune-boosting nutrients like antioxidants and immunity-boosting minerals and vitamins. Plus, protein is also actively involved in healing and recovery after an illness.

Simply put, our immune cells consist of proteins, and we need optimum protein in our diet to be able to resist and chase away unwanted intruders.

## Are You Eating Enough?

It's a sad truth that many of us don't get enough protein and are deficient in this life-saving nutrient. The common signs of protein deficiency are sluggish metabolism, loss of muscle mass, low energy levels and fatigue, and a general feeling of unexplained tiredness, foggy brain, poor concentration, moodiness, mood swings, muscle, bone and joint pain, slow wound healing and low immunity.

It is important to keep a look out for these signs.

## Who Is at Risk?

Today, many of us are at risk of protein deficiency, especially growing teenagers, fitness enthusiasts and athletes who exercise regularly as they burn more calories and use more protein to build muscle. Another group at risk is that of pregnant and lactating women since their biological needs are heightened. Vegetarians and vegans are also among those who don't get enough complete protein since plant-based protein sources are limited and, at times, difficult to access.

The elderly can also be at risk of deficiency if their diet is not modified to serve their needs because as we age, our digestion and ability to use protein gets less efficient. To heal, you need at least one and a half times the normal protein recommendations; therefore, those recovering from an acute illness or injury need to keep a strict check on their protein intake. Since stress hormones increase muscle and tissue breakdown in times of both physical and emotional stress, those suffering additional stress must also watch out for protein deficiency. If you're on a weight-loss diet, adequate protein is needed to balance blood sugars and prevent muscle breakdown. For those with digestive issues or low stomach acid, a protein-rich diet will help balance the acid production in the stomach and lead to better digestion. Certain trends show that women tend to have a lower protein intake compared to men; therefore, they need to increase the number of protein sources in their diet.

In fact, even if you don't fall in any of the above categories, it still pays to make sure that your protein intake is adequate.

## How Much Is Enough?

The right amount of protein for a person depends on many factors—their activity levels, age, muscle mass, physique goals and current state of health. Usually, a common formula used is 0.8 grams of protein per kilogram of ideal body weight. For example, an average man weighing 70 kilograms would require 56 grams of protein per day and a woman weighing 60 kilograms would need about 48 grams of protein per day. Another simple way to determine our protein needs is to eat approximately the number of grams per inch of your height. For example if your height is 65 inches, target 65 grams of protein per day.

Eating a balanced diet can help us get enough protein in our diet. But there are rules:

- It important to focus on both the quantity and the quality of protein. Not all food sources of protein contain all the nine essential amino acids our body requires. In fact, many vegetarian proteins (cereals and lentils) are incomplete proteins as some amino acids are missing. And since the majority of the protein in Indian diets comes from vegetarian sources, our diets tend to be predominantly low in quality protein. Therefore, look closely at your plate to check whether you are eating enough high-quality complete protein (with all essential amino acids) or not.
- Opt for leaner protein options over high-fat versions. Plant-based protein, such as beans, nuts and seeds are great options, as are lean meats, low-fat dairy, eggs and fish. Try to include one good protein source in every meal of the day.
- Score enough of the amino acid cysteine. It is found in most high-protein foods, such as chicken, turkey, yoghurt, cheese, eggs, sunflower seeds and legumes.

**Fun Fact:** Our blood is red because of a protein, haemoglobin, that carries oxygen from the lungs to the body's cells and disposes of harmful waste products like carbon dioxide.

# 18

# Eat Good Fats

'What's a good fat? Fat is fat, right? And it's bad for us,' I am told by people very often. And that's my cue to begin a tutorial to explain the different kinds of fats and their importance on every aspect of our health.

Fats add taste to food. Almost everyone will vouch for that. Yet for years, fat has been getting a bad rap to the extent that when we hear the word 'fat', we automatically think 'bad' and are constantly on a hunt for fat-free foods.

Thankfully, now we have a more progressive attitude towards dietary fat, and the new advice going around is that 'fat is okay, but you have to eat the right kind'. Although fats are not considered harmful anymore, that is not a go-ahead for overeating butter or wolfing down cheeseburgers; instead, it is a mandate for fish, nuts and switching to good, healthy oils.

The key is to separate the good from the bad. Yes, not all fats are created equal. Some fats increase our risk of heart disease while some promote our health positively.

### Good to Know

There is no license to add fat to the diet willy-nilly. Too much total fat—more than about 25 per cent of calories—is still a bad idea. And adding a small amount of good fats to an unhealthy diet does not work. In fact, good fat works best when it replaces bad fat or carbohydrates. As a general rule, keep the overall level of fats low and ensure that most of this is made up of good fats.

## The Effects

Dietary fats supply some of the best and most stable sources of energy. So, if you want to feel good all day long, you need to eat enough and only the right types of fat. Essential fatty acids are needed for good, shiny hair, healthy skin and strong joints. We need them for proper hormone production, an imbalance of which may cause problems like premenstrual syndrome (PMS), or other hormonal aberrations. Besides, if hormone production is off, your metabolism, which has a direct bearing on your weight, will follow suit. And yes it is needed for stronger immunty too.

## The Immunity Connection

Vitamins A, D, E and K, which are essential, immunity-boosting nutrients are fat-soluble, that is, we need fats to absorb these vitamins into our body. Medium-chain fatty acids (MCFAs) like those present in coconut oil help with the absorption of antioxidants and other nutrients from food (yes, that's why cooking in coconut oil every now and then is a good idea). Similarly, adding a dressing to a salad helps increase the absorption of fat-soluble vitamins from vegetables and fruits. It turns out that the body needs a little bit of fat to digest these vitamins and the same goes for countless antioxidants too that we hope to receive from vegetables.

Fat is needed to create hormones in the body, including prostaglandins, which help control blood pressure, cut inflammation and modulate the immune response. Fat is found around almost all tissues in our body and has its own immune system. There are special guardian immune cells, called adipose type one innate lymphoid cells (ILCs), which keep macrophages in check, and guard against inflammation and metabolic disease that could happen when the number of macrophages increases.

Fatty acids are potent modulators of the immune response. Conjugated linoleic acid available in meat and dairy products stimulates the immune system and prevents breast cancer.

Excess unhealthy oil in your diet may impair the WBCs, which fight off infections. In addition, high-fat diets can negatively impact gut microbiota, which helps your immune system stay strong. Yes, the kind of fat you eat can drastically change the kind of bacteria that live in the intestines, which directly impacts the immune system.

---

## TO-DO

Our immune system is particularly sensitive to both the amount and the types of fats we eat. Excess fat (any kind) in the diet depresses the immune system, makes it lazy and puts it to sleep. It also suppresses the activity of the natural killer cells and leads to the formation of inflammation-causing free radicals. Thus, with fat, low to moderate is the way to go.

- It is important to replace bad fats with good fats and keep it to 20–25 per cent of your total calorie intake for the day, of which only 10 per cent should come from saturated fats.

- It makes sense to focus on consuming essential fatty acids (EFA's) as our body cannot make them indigenously because, like vitamins, minerals and other essential nutrients, we must get them from the foods we eat.
- Let us now look at a few good fat options that you can include in your diet.

**Ghee**

Now that we know that saturated fat is not the devil it was considered to be; it's time to get a little ghee back in our diet. It is now clear that excess carbohydrates and sugar in our diet are more to be blamed for obesity than saturated fat. So go on, smear a little ghee on the roti, or add some tempering to your curry without fear.

**Fatty Fish**

There is no doubt that omega-3 fatty acids have the amazing power to keep the body free of heart disease and diabetes. They also play a significant role in fending off increasingly common illnesses like asthma, arthritis, depression, rheumatoid arthritis and even certain types of cancer. You need to put more of this wonder nutrient on your plate. Fatty fish such as salmon, tuna, sardines, mackerel and trout are the richest sources of omega-3. So, make sure you eat these foods at least twice a week.

**Flaxseeds**

If you hate fish or are a strict vegetarian, add flaxseeds to your diet for a boost of alpha-linolenic acid (which gets converted to omega-3 fatty acid in the body). Have one tablespoon of flaxseeds three to four times a week (sprinkle on soups, curries, dals), or incorporate some flaxseed oil in your cooking.

## Nuts

How can foods so high in fat be good for your health? Well, that's because most of the fats found in nuts are unsaturated fats. Almonds, for example, pack in lots of monounsaturated fatty acids (MUFA), which are great for our heart as they help lower bad cholesterol, LDL and increase HDL, the good cholesterol. Walnuts, besides MUFA, also have omega-3 that helps lower cholesterol levels, reduce inflammation and improve blood flow through the arteries. Don't forget to grab a few nuts every day.

## Nut butters

These are a good way of harnessing the health benefits that nuts offer. Peanut, walnut, almond or cashew butter are good options that deliver good quality protein along with good fats. Just read the labels carefully and opt for butters that don't have added sugars or you could make your own at home.

## Coconut

Coconut is loaded with saturated fat, which is why it was considered bad for the arteries and was shunned for a long time. But now we know that it is heart-healthy because more than 50 per cent of it is lauric acid, a compound that actually boosts HDL (good) cholesterol and helps decrease the risk of heart disease. So, add some coconut in your curries or munch on some as a snack.

## Eggs

One whole egg contains 5 grams of fat, but only 1.5 grams are saturated fat. Whole eggs are also a good source of choline (one egg yolk has about 300 micrograms of choline), an important nutrient that helps regulate the brain, nervous system and cardiovascular system. And while there's much buzz about the cholesterol in eggs, moderate egg consumption is actually linked to improved heart health.

# 19

# The Important Vitamins

Science and research often confuse us more instead of providing a satisfactory explanation. Theories change at an alarming rate. But thankfully, one fact that has stood steadfast is that vitamins are essential for our health and for us to function at an optimum level. Another fact that has become increasingly clear over the years is that they have a huge say in our immunity. Unfortunately, information about the same is not understood too well.

## Score Vitamin A

Vitamin A is an imperative immunity-boosting vitamin and unfortunately, its deficiency is widespread too, so is a lack of information about foods rich in it. For example, while kale is universally lauded as a superfood loaded with vitamin A, not many know that our humble, easily accessible sweet potato delivers just as much vitamin A. It's time to change the status quo and make all sources of vitamins accessible.

### Know the Vitamin

Vitamin A is a broad group of related nutrients and includes retinoids delivered from animal sources (like retinol), carotenoids (alpha, beta, gamma and zeta carotenes) and xanthophylls (astaxanthin, lutein, zeaxanthin and many more) from plant sources. The most common carotene is beta carotene and our body converts it into vitamin A.

All these compounds work together to ensure that our eyes stay sharp, the reproductive system at its efficient best, bones strong and immunity in good shape.

## The Immunity Connection

Vitamin A is also known as an anti-inflammation vitamin and thus has a significant role in enhancing the immune function of our body. It is an antioxidant too; it helps prevent the cells from getting damaged due to oxidative stress. Continual cell damage from oxidative stress can lead to chronic diseases.

It protects the immune system by strengthening WBCs production and increasing the immune function by supporting the growth and distribution of T-cells.

Vitamin A helps grow, maintain and strengthen epithelium and mucous tissues that line the majority of our organs. These tissues are the body's first line of defence against pathogens and are an important part of our body's immune response to infection.

It has a particularly profound effect on the gut mucosal immune system and helps increase antimicrobial peptides to defeat the pathogens. Vitamin A is the key to the gut making all the right decisions. Its deficiency can throw our immunity out of gear.

In addition, vitamin A is needed to maintain the mucosal barriers of the innate (the one we are born with) immune system. Thus, its deficiency can compromise the integrity of this first line of defence, thereby increasing susceptibility to some types of infection like eye, gastrointestinal and respiratory tract.

# TO-DO

- The human body cannot synthesize vitamin A; it must be absorbed by the intestine from the diet.
- Sweet potatoes are the best source of carotenoids (yes, they are higher than carrots). You can also target spinach for xanthophylls and shrimps or eggs for retinoids.
- You can also get it from carrots and other red, yellow, orange and dark-green leafy vegetables like spinach, red peppers, mango, sweet potato, pumpkin and broccoli.

**Good to Know**
Vitamin A is a fat-soluble vitamin.
So it is essential to add some good
fats to your diet.

Beta carotene is not a very heat-sensitive
nutrient, so cooking the foods lightly
will not destroy it.

**Fun Fact:** Marguerite Davis and Elmer Verner McCollum, two American biochemists, co-discovered the existence of vitamin A in 1913.

## Get Enough Vitamin C

Who doesn't have a childhood memory of biting into a tangy, sweet guava and gaining immeasurable happiness out of it? Almost everyone I know does. Some lucky ones even remember plucking slightly raw ones off the tress and eating them with abandon, almost as a metaphor of free, uncluttered living.

But why are we talking about guava here? Apart from the feel-good factor, guavas are a gold mine of nutrients and provide a lot of vitamin C, even more than the other popular source—oranges. And we need enough vitamin C to keep our immunity at its optimum level.

## Know the Vitamin

The importance of getting enough vitamin C is a no-brainer. Besides its effect on our immunity, it is an important antioxidant too, meaning it neutralizes free radicals generated in the body due to exposure to environmental stressors like UV exposure, pollution, etc. Free radicals are charged particles that trigger harmful inflammation and damage cells, tissues and our genes if left unchecked.

Vitamin C is also required for the growth and repair of tissues in the body and is important for the absorption of iron, which is necessary to combat fatigue and exhaustion.

## The Immunity Connection

Vitamin C's connection with immunity is straightforward and works on multiple levels. This key antioxidant acts as an immune enhancer by helping WBCs perform at their peak.

It quickens the immune system's response time and increases the levels of interferon—an antibody which coats cell surfaces and is responsible for preventing the entry of viruses. Additionally, vitamin C supports the production and activity of antibodies, and good antibody function is vital for a healthy immune system.

Vitamin C also enhances the function of phagocytes, the WBCs that surround pathogens and other dangerous particles, and digest and neutralize them enzymatically.

When foreign particles infiltrate the body, vitamin C helps

direct immune cells called neutrophils to the site of infection and defend these cells against free radicals.

Vitamin C also helps strengthen the fatty membranes in the skin and the connective tissue and thus helps protect organs like the lungs from pathogens.

It also helps to activate several key enzymes in the body, which synthesize hormones that help build collagen—an essential protein in skin that we need for proper wound healing. And as our skin is our first line of defence, an injury on the skin, if not rectified quickly, can become a doorway for infection-causing bacteria.

Similarly, the adrenal glands also play a key role in our body's response to stress, and they too use a significant amount of vitamin C each time a stress response gets triggered.

### Good to Know
The common signs of vitamin C deficiency one must look out for are weak immunity, weak bones, infections, skin problems, poor wound healing, joint pain, depression, fatigue, inflammation, bleeding gums, scurvy and anaemia.

Finally, vitamin C alone cannot fight this tough battle for us. To have a strong immune system, the diet must contain ample antioxidants, micro-nutrients and all essential vitamins and minerals.

---

### TO-DO

Our body can't make its own vitamin C or store the nutrient efficiently, as this water-soluble vitamin dissolves once ingested and is excreted in the urine. So it is vital to get the daily requirement through food every day.

The good news is that vitamin C is present in so many foods that you don't need to take a vitamin C supplement, nor do you need to restrict yourself to only guavas and oranges. Include a few foods that I've mentioned below in your diet every day to make sure you get enough of this essential vitamin.

- Eat two guavas daily to more than meet your vitamin C needs.
- Amla is the most underrated berry around. An amla a day is enough for your daily vitamin C requirement. You can even juice it, or grate some into your soups and stir-fries. If sweet is your poison, then go for some amla murabba or amla candy.
- A delightful, crisp and easy-to-eat vegetable named shankhalu in West Bengal (also called yam bean or jicama) is also loaded with vitamin C. It is high in fibre and is a perfect addition to salads.
- Cape gooseberries (rasbhari) are really tangy (many find them downright sour), so you might need to develop a taste for it. This is something I earnestly advise because they are loaded with vitamin C.
- Lobia (black-eyed peas or black-eyed beans) have a decent amount of vitamin C too, besides lots of fibre and protein. So please look beyond its more popular cousins—rajma and chickpea—and maybe have a lobia and cucumber salad today.
- Lychees are delicious, and this sweetest of all fruits delivers vitamin C too, besides providing multiple electrolytes that are hard to find. As this exotic fruit has a very short shelf life (and so is available for a very limited time even during its season), have it when it is available.

- Raw bananas and plantain have a good amount of vitamin C, plus vitamin A (in plantains). They are also good sources of potassium and vitamin B6.
- Think purple and go for the fabulous, tongue-coating, dark java plum (better known as jamun in India). It gives a considerable amount of vitamin C for very few calories.
- While tamarind is a rich source of iron, it is also packed with vitamin C. Use it liberally in your curries and chutneys.
- Amaranth (chollai ka saag) has vitamin C in abundance.
- Look beyond greens and eat your reds too, namely, red cabbage and beets. One cup of chopped crimson will not just add about 50 milligrams of vitamin C, but is also full of phytochemicals and flavonoids.
- Papaya is an often-overlooked source of vitamin C. Have a quarter plate a day and your stomach will thank you. It'll also help clear up your sinuses.
- If you like them exotic, then kiwis, strawberries and pineapple are all fantastic sources of vitamin C.
- Some more sources of vitamin C are:
  - Bell peppers (yellow, red and green)
  - Broccoli
  - Lemon
  - Lime (mausambi)
  - Strawberries
  - Cauliflower
  - Cabbage
  - Mustard greens
  - Kohlrabi
  - Tomatoes
  - Mango
  - Green chilli

## Boost Its Absorption!

Vitamin C is a very sensitive nutrient that reacts to air, water and heat, so it is best consumed via raw foods. Similarly, thawing and freezing vegetables over a long period may also lead to the loss of vitamin C.

**Good to Know**

Smokers tend to be deficient in vitamin C,
as their body uses it in excess to detoxify.
So, smokers need more vitamin C.

## Avoid the Supplement!

Before you reach out for vitamin C tablets to ward off a cold or score more of this vitamin, please know that most of the time, vitamin C supplements contain an excess amount of the vitamin, and our body will usually end up excreting it through urine. Also, it's easy to get recommended amounts without popping a pill. Just focus on including vitamin C foods in your daily diet.

**Fun Fact:** The importance of vitamin C, also known as ascorbic acid, was first realized more than 250 years ago when its deficiency was discovered to be the cause of scurvy.

## Put the Spotlight on Vitamin E

It is increasingly getting clear that eating a diet with enough energy and nutrients, both macro and micro, may no longer be enough to save us from modern ailments and bless us with a disease-free, long life. This is due to the toxic, polluted times we live in and the onslaught of stress we struggle with every day. What we need today are sources that deliver a large dose of antioxidants and anti-inflammatory agents—vitamin E is one such agent.

## Know the Vitamin

This fat-soluble vitamin present in many foods, especially certain fats and oils, is a powerful antioxidant (similar in function to other better-known antioxidants like vitamin C and beta-carotene) that protects cells in the body from damage caused by free radicals. Highly reactive substances, free radicals are formed as a result of metabolism in the body and from exposure to factors in the environment like cigarette smoke and ultraviolet light. They cause damage to body cells and contribute to the development of health issues like heart disease and cancer.

## The Immunity Connection

Vitamin E is found in higher concentrations in immune cells compared to other cells in the blood and is an important nutrient for immune function modulation. It is part of nearly 200 biochemical reactions in your body and is critical for immune system functions.

Vitamin E helps boost levels of T-lymphocytes or T-cells. It also helps these cells multiply correctly and communicate with other immune processes. And as T-cells decrease with age, maintaining optimal intake of vitamin E is essential for an efficient immune system.

Vitamin E is an antioxidant; so it helps prevent the free radicals caused due to oxidative stress in the body from damaging the cells. Free radicals bind to cells in a way that causes damage to the protein and DNA inside. Vitamin E helps neutralize this threat.

*Spot the Deficiency*

Signs of vitamin E deficiency include weak muscles, fertility issues, abnormal eye movements, impaired vision and unsteady gait.

Vitamin E deficiency is very rare, but can happen if an extremely low-fat diet is followed for a prolonged period (serial dieters, beware!). The deficiency is also seen in people who are unable to absorb fat properly due to conditions like pancreatitis (inflammation of the pancreas), cystic fibrosis and biliary diseases (illnesses of the gallbladder and biliary ducts).

*The Benefits Are Many*

Vitamin E is our skin's best friend. It acts as a natural anti-aging nutrient and also protects the skin from ultraviolet radiation. Similarly, it is great for our hair as it helps decrease environmental damage and promotes circulation in the scalp.

It helps stave off heart disease by preventing the arteries from clogging and forming blood clots that could lead to a heart attack. It also thins the blood and helps lower blood pressure.

**Good to Know**

Vitamin E helps ease menopause, has an antioxidant action and is great for our muscle health too.
It helps ease muscle aches and aids in muscle repair after a tough workout.

- Vitamin E is a fat-soluble vitamin. This means the body doesn't need it every day as any excess is stored for future use.
- It occurs naturally in eight different forms, including four tocopherols (alpha, beta, gamma and delta) and four tocotrienols. Alpha-tocopherol is the most common and most potent form of the vitamin.
- To maximize your vitamin E intake, eat a diet peppered with foods such as wheat germ, liver, eggs, chicken, turkey, salmon, mackerel, nuts (almonds, hazelnuts and walnuts), sunflower seeds, cold-pressed vegetable oils, including olive, corn, safflower, soybean, cottonseed and canola. Fruits like apples, apricots, peaches, dark green leafy vegetables like spinach and broccoli, and other veggies like beet, turnip sweet potatoes, yams and sprouts should also be included.

### Good to Know

If you smoke, consume high amounts of alcohol, or don't exercise much, you are probably in dire need to particularly boost your vitamin E intake

**Fun Fact:** Biological activity of natural vitamin E (from food) is three times more than that of synthetic vitamin E.

20

# The Important Minerals

Micronutrient malnutrition, in which a person is deficient in some essential vitamins and trace minerals, is the most overlooked and thus is the most dangerous kind of deficiency which can undermine our health and our immunity in particular. And here, the detection of deficiencies of the trace minerals that our body needs in minuscule amounts gets missed the most.

## The Underdog of Immunity—Selenium

If this is the first time you've read about selenium—don't worry, it's not your fault. There is not much known about this trace mineral out there. But that doesn't mean it is not important. In fact, like any fighting force, healthy immune system warriors need good, regular nourishment, and selenium is one such trace mineral that they need to stay fighting fit.

### Know the Mineral

Selenium is involved in processes throughout the body, starting in the brain down to the tips of our toes. It is needed to keep our metabolism and thyroid function active. It supports cognitive function and is a potent antioxidant that helps lower oxidative stress, which has been linked to many chronic diseases, from type 2 diabetes to some types of cancer.

Its deficiency is connected to depression, thyroid malfunction—since selenium concentration is higher in the thyroid gland than in any other organ in the body—infertility and weakened immunity.

## The Immunity Connection

Selenium's ability to lower oxidative damage does more than just boost our heart's health. It also helps lower inflammation and strengthen the immune system. In simple words, selenium deficiency may actually slow down immune cell response.

This trace mineral boosts the antioxidant power of vitamin E and is also vital for the production of the two most powerful antioxidant and anti-aging enzymes in the body—superoxide dismutase (SOD) and glutathione peroxidase.

In fact, selenium and antioxidants that boost our immunity and fight inflammation go well together. Selenium functions as a cofactor for antioxidant enzymes that protect our tissues from oxidative damage. This mineral also increases WBC count and is needed for the proper functioning of important immune cells like neutrophils, macrophages, natural killer cells, T-lymphocytes and other immune mechanisms. Selenium deficiency is known to impair antibody production in the body.

Finally it also helps our body efficiently utilize vitamin C, a known immunity booster. Although this super-mineral does not get as much press as calcium and iron, it is more important for our immunity than you may have previously thought.

**Good to Know**
Selenium deficiency often leads to muscle weakness and pain, hair loss and mental fog.

Excess selenium in your body can lead to nausea, vomiting, abdominal pain, dermatitis, nail abnormalities, fatigue, irritability, impaired endocrine function, neurotoxicity and weight loss. This condition is rare, but one can avoid it by sticking to food sources and abstaining from arbitrary supplementation.

---

### TO-DO

- The important thing to know is that as we cannot produce selenium ourselves, we have to rely on our diet for its supply. This is as easy as including a few foods that are known sources of selenium, such as meat, seafood, eggs and dairy products in our daily or weekly diet.
- If you are a vegetarian or a vegan, then you too have enough options to choose from. Chickpeas, kidney beans, nuts (especially pine nuts, Brazil nuts, peanuts, cashew and almonds) seeds like chia, pumpkin and sunflower, dark chocolate, brown rice, wheat germ, whole grains, asparagus, broccoli, spinach, zucchini and mushrooms are good plant-based sources of selenium. Garlic, peaches and banana also deliver some selenium.

**Good to Know**
A single Brazil nut provides enough
to meet the daily requirement of selenium
for a human adult.

**Fun Fact:** Selenium gets its name from the Greek word 'selene,' which means 'moon.' Selene was the Greek goddess of the moon.

---

# Get the Zinc Zing

A sick child's refusal to swallow a pill led to the discovery of one of zinc's most interesting applications as a cure for the common cold. Instead of swallowing a zinc tablet, the little girl in question let it melt in her mouth. To her father's surprise, her cold symptoms disappeared within hours. Since then, of course, it has been established beyond doubt how critical zinc is for healthy body functioning and how, without it, 300 critical enzymes in our body will cease to function.

## Know the Mineral

So, what does this trace nutrient do? Zinc is essential for reading genetic instructions, and your diet does not contain enough zinc; instructions get misread or downright ignored, leading to malfunctions in the body. Zinc is also involved in the metabolism of proteins, carbohydrates and lipids in the body. It helps support optimum blood sugar balance. Without enough zinc, the insulin response decreases and it becomes more difficult to stabilize our blood sugar.

With zinc in our diet, the absorption of minerals by our body increases. By helping the body absorb calcium better, it helps prevent osteoporosis. Zinc is needed by the liver to function properly, and also for bone mineralization, proper thyroid function and sperm production. Attention, memory, problem-solving and hand-eye coordination—all improve with zinc.

Zinc is also needed by our body to help prevent acne. Since it's essential for tissue growth and repair across the body, it's instrumental in accelerating wound healing. It promotes hair growth as it is an essential ingredient in melanin, which is the natural pigment in hair.

Kavita Devgan

Gustin is a small protein that is directly involved in our sense of taste. Zinc works along with gustin to let our sense of taste function properly.

## The Immunity Connection

This mineral's nutritional importance has been known for a long time, but its importance for immunity modulation has come into the limelight in the last few decades. In fact, now we know that maintaining our zinc levels optimizes the functioning of our immune system and could be a key to living a long, healthier life.

Zinc activates enzymes that break down proteins in viruses and bacteria to stop their spread. It also repels the viruses from attaching to our cells. It's known to fight off microbes like streptococcus pneumonia, a type of bacteria that causes the dangerous lung disease, pneumonia. Zinc can block the pathway these bacteria use to take in nutrients, essentially starving the bacteria and making it easier for your immune cells to kill them.

It helps avoid infections by preventing out-of-control inflammation in the body that can be damaging and even deadly. Zinc helps fight off a range of viral infections—from herpes to common cold, especially respiratory infections. It can help block the cold virus from replicating and spreading throughout the body.

This mineral is needed for the production and optimal functioning of immune cells, like T-cells and WBCs, that help the body fight off diseases. In fact, the growth or function of the immune cells like macrophages, neutrophils, natural killer cells, T-cells and B-cell can get impaired by zinc deficiency.

Zinc can have a positive effect on gut lining and help prevent leaky gut syndrome (a condition where loose gaps in the intestinal wall allow harmful substances such as bacteria and other toxins to pass through into the bloodstream), which is a known cause of widespread inflammation that often downs our immunity system.

Zinc is actually the gatekeeper of the immune system. So, to score a healthy immunity, ensure enough zinc intake in the diet.

## Check the Signs

The first signs of zinc deficiency are impairment of taste, a poor immune response and skin problems. Other symptoms of zinc deficiency include hair loss, diarrhoea, frequent cold and infections, fatigue, delayed wound healing and growth failure in children.

## How Much Do We Need?

Zinc is a micromineral needed in the diet on a daily basis, but only in minimal amounts. Moderate intake of zinc, approximately 8 to 11 milligrams daily, is adequate to prevent deficiencies.

**Good to Know**

Regular alcohol drinkers also tend to have zinc deficiency as alcohol decreases zinc absorption from our diet and increases the loss of zinc in urine.

During pregnancy, the requirements are higher as zinc deficiency may slow foetal development. Breastfeeding women must also include a generous serving of at least one good source of zinc in their diet each day. Those suffering from anaemia generally need higher amounts of zinc in their diet than an average person.

The recommended amount of zinc for adult men is higher than that for women. Men need more zinc than women because male semen contains 100 times more zinc than is found in the blood.

Age is a factor too. Elderly people also need to maintain an adequate zinc status to prevent a weaker immune system, particularly against pneumonia. For those not eating an optimal diet to strengthen their immune function, immunity begins to diminish around the age of 60 to 65. But even those who are eating a proper diet may need zinc supplements.

A vegetarian diet often contains less zinc than a meat-based diet and so it is essential for vegetarians to eat plenty of rich sources. Zinc requirements are estimated to be about 50 per cent higher for vegetarians due to reduced bioavailability from plant foods.

Phytate, an antioxidant compound found in whole grains, legumes, nuts and seeds, prevents the absorption of certain minerals, including zinc. In addition, other minerals such as iron and calcium interfere with zinc absorption. Copper also competes with zinc for binding proteins inside the body's cells. So be careful about excess supplementation of these minerals.

## Too Much Is Too Bad

There is something called too much zinc. Don't go for arbitrary supplementation, as excess zinc can be toxic, and too much zinc interferes with the absorption and metabolism of other minerals in the body, particularly iron and copper, and actually weakens immunity. Copper deficiency can lead to lower numbers of WBCs, and it can also negatively affect immune cells due to which we might face a harder time fighting off an illness.

- Zinc deficiency is probably a bigger problem than most people realize. Preventing that deficiency is important. With zinc, consistency is key. Foods rich in zinc must be included daily in the diet to score enough.
- The richest source of zinc are oysters, but you can get a fair share via seafood, chicken, lamb and turkey. Vegetarian sources such as yoghurt, eggs, seeds (pumpkin, sesame and watermelon), nuts (cashews, pine nuts, almonds and peanuts), whole grains (oats and wheat germ), tofu, legumes (kidney beans, chickpeas), some vegetables like spinach, mushrooms, zucchini and broccoli also deliver zinc but in lower amounts.

*Tip: Combine dry fruits like almonds, walnuts, raisins and cashews along with seeds like sunflower seeds, pumpkin seeds, hemp seeds and sesame seeds into a trail mix. Use this mix as a snack or as salad garnishing, desserts and cereals.*

**Good to Know**

Zinc from breast milk is better absorbed than that from formula milk. Colostrum, the first milk produced by the mother, is loaded with zinc.

**Fun Fact:** Zinc is the second most abundant metal in the human body, after iron.

## The Magnesium Connection

There is a powerful mineral that keeps working in the background and doesn't get much press, which is why not many know about it. This silent saviour is magnesium.

The truth is that almost no system, organ or process in the body can function without enough magnesium. It is omnipresent—found everywhere from bones, to muscles and soft tissues, with trace amounts circulating in the blood as well. In fact, a lesser-known important fact is that magnesium deficiency is the most common deficiency worldwide after vitamin D.

It's time to pay attention to magnesium.

## Know the Mineral

When you are stressed, magnesium is the first mineral that is depleted from the body. Magnesium alleviates stress, allowing you to relax and fall asleep. It activates over 300 enzyme reactions in the body, which in turn, affect thousands of essential processes happening inside the body at any moment.

Magnesium is beneficial for the nervous system. Our nerves require this mineral to send and receive messages. It is the most crucial mineral needed for muscle contraction and relaxation, and its deficiency can lead to muscle cramps, aches and pains. It is also needed for blood coagulation, nutrient metabolism and energy production. Are you constantly feeling tired? You might have a magnesium deficiency.

A lack of magnesium can raise blood pressure and reduce insulin sensitivity. Those with respiratory diseases such as asthma need to be particularly careful about their magnesium intake since it helps relax the muscles of the bronchioles in the lungs. Magnesium also plays a crucial role in our immune response.

## The Immunity Connection

Magnesium acts as a cofactor (a substance that helps chemical reactions occur) for various immune system reactions.

Secondly, magnesium deficiency correlates with higher levels of inflammation in the body. When you are magnesium-deficient, WBCs get activated and release inflammatory chemicals in the body. In fact, enough magnesium in the diet helps decrease the levels of C-reactive protein (CRP) in the blood, which is a marker of inflammation.

Thirdly, low magnesium levels can lead to low levels of vitamin D, as magnesium acts as a cofactor in the vitamin D activation reactions in the liver and kidneys and is essential for its metabolism. We have already established the importance of vitamin D in boosting immunity.

Last but not least, it is really important to know in today's angst-ridden times that healthy magnesium levels protect against depression since magnesium is important for the release and binding of serotonin, the happy hormone in the brain. And staying happy and stress-free is a prerequisite for good immunity.

## Are You Deficient?

It is actually challenging to find out if one has a magnesium deficiency, as blood tests aren't very dependable. Another catch is that the symptoms of magnesium deficiency—muscle cramps, facial and eye tics, poor sleep, hyperactivity, and chronic pain—are similar to the symptoms of other deficiencies, particularly vitamin B12 and vitamin D.

**Good to Know**
Constipation, frequent headaches,
restless legs syndrome and kidney stones are some
other tell-tale signs.

So, our best bet is to prevent deficiency and consciously ensure that there is enough magnesium in our diets. Ensuring enough magnesium in the diet is a straightforward strategy to score healthy immunity.

## TO-DO

Our body needs about 400 milligrams of magnesium daily. The densest sources of this mineral are dark leafy greens, especially spinach, nuts (particularly almonds, walnuts, cashews and peanuts), seeds (especially pumpkin seeds and sunflower seeds), fish (mackerel, salmon and halibut) beans, whole grains, avocados, yoghurt, bananas, dried fruit, eggplant and unsweetened cocoa.

A sample diet featuring enough magnesium will include:

- Spinach 250 gm (200 mg) or mackerel 250 gm (200 mg),
- 1 tablespoon or about 10 grams pumpkin seeds (60 mg)
- 2 cups yoghurt (100 mg)
- 10 almonds (30 mg)
- 1 banana (30 mg)

*Be Careful*

While eating the right foods is important, avoiding the wrong ones is equally important. Most dark-coloured sodas contain phosphates, which bind with magnesium inside our digestive tract and make it unavailable to the body. Antacids disrupt magnesium absorption, and excessive sugar, caffeine and alcohol cause the body to excrete magnesium through the kidneys.

Chronic stress is a big villain and affects the body in myriad ways, one of which is that it can magnify magnesium deficiency. Therefore, it is essential that we learn to curb and manage stress. Those who take diuretics, birth control pills, insulin and frequent antibiotics need to be careful too as such medications lead to magnesium leaching from the body. And if you pop calcium pills frequently, be aware that calcium supplementation can lead to the depletion of magnesium in your body, so add a magnesium supplement to your routine as well.

> **Fun Fact**: About 60 per cent of magnesium in the body is found in the skeleton, 39 per cent in the muscles and 1 per cent is extracellular.

## Get Iron Power

Iron deficiency is the most common nutritional deficiency worldwide, and if left untreated, it can result in health issues like fatigue and anaemia. Iron deficiency is like a silent assassin that slowly but surely messes up our health from the inside, and its prolonged deficiency can prove to be extremely debilitating, as this mineral is vital to our body, fitness and overall well-being.

### How Do You Know You Are Deficient?

As far as iron deficiency is concerned, blood tests are a reliable tool to understand the levels in your blood. Ferritin is a protein that helps us store iron safely in the blood, so it is a good marker for the amount of iron in the body. Haemoglobin levels are another standard indicator.

**Good to Know**

The deficiency symptoms to look out for are:

- Unexplained fatigue and general weakness
- Dizziness
- Sensitivity to cold
- Shortness of breath even after light physical activity (say, climbing stairs)
- Pica (cravings for ice or non-food items)

*Know the Mineral*

In food, iron is present in two different forms: heme iron and non-heme iron. The way our body absorbs these two types of iron is very different. Heme iron, found in eggs, meat, fish, and poultry, is easily absorbed and used by our body. Non-heme iron, on the other hand, is found in vegetarian sources like tofu, beans and legumes, fruits and vegetables, dark leafy greens—mainly spinach and kale and iron-fortified cereals and supplements. Non-heme iron is more difficult to absorb.

This is one reason why vegetarians, even if their diet includes dairy and eggs, are at a higher risk of developing an iron deficiency than people who eat meat.

*Why We Need Iron*

Iron is ubiquitous in nature and is present in every cell. We need it for strength and vigour, and it plays a key role in DNA and enzyme synthesis and multiple basic life processes in the body.

Iron is an important component of haemoglobin, a protein molecule that transports oxygen throughout the body to the lung, tissues, brain and muscles. In fact, about 70 per cent of iron in the body is found in red blood cells, and iron deficiency can lead to anaemia—a common disorder in which a dearth of iron leads to pallid skin, dizziness and shortness of breath—which occurs when the blood does not carry enough oxygen to the body.

In addition, iron plays a vital role in brain function, particularly in learning and memory, and when our body is deficient in iron, we tend to gain weight. Yes, while you become pale and weak on the outside, your weight may actually increase. For those with an iron deficiency, adequate oxygen cannot reach the cells as iron is a building block of haemoglobin, the carrier of oxygen to different parts of the body; this leads to severe metabolism slowdown, which translates to lesser calories burnt and thus more fat stored in the body. Besides, the fatigue and listlessness that often accompany iron deficiency lead to skipping exercise, which can play a role in weight gain.

## The Immune Connection

Enough iron in the diet is essential for proper functioning of the immune system and to help the body fight infections. One of the signs of being iron-deficient is that you fall sick very often and for longer period.

When haemoglobin is low and oxygen supply is affected, the organs get affected and immunity takes a huge hit. Iron is necessary for the proliferation and maturation of immune cells, particularly lymphocytes.

---

## TO-DO

### Get Your Fill

To go from deficient to optimized, get your fill of iron by regularly putting lean meat, liver, fortified cereal and soy nuts on your plate. Fresh fruits like prunes, pomegranate, watermelon and figs also have iron, as do dried varieties of raisins, apricots, dates and peaches.

### Boost Iron Absorption Consciously

- Some foods like whole grains, soy, nuts, spinach, beets and legumes contain phytates that can decrease the amount of non-heme iron absorbed from the food. So try to pair these with those foods that enhance non-heme absorption! For example, dress your greens with a homemade, orange or lemon juice based dressing to enhance non-heme absorption, as vitamin C found in oranges and lemons helps boost the absorption. Or throw in some tomatoes or other vitamin C rich foods like broccoli, bell pepper, strawberries, citrus fruits, papaya, cauliflower, amla (gooseberry) for better iron absorption.
- Excess intake of some minerals like zinc, magnesium, calcium and copper can inhibit non-heme iron absorption. So if you take supplements of these minerals, take them a few hours before or after mealtime. Similarly, consider having your glass of calcium-rich milk a couple of hours before or after your iron-rich meal.
- Increase the gap between your coffee/tea and breakfast. Don't have these two things side-by-side as tannins and polyphenols—the compounds present in tea and coffee—can inhibit iron absorption. These compounds can bind with iron, therefore making non-heme iron insoluble. Be sure to leave a couple of hours between your non-heme iron-rich lunch and your afternoon tea. Avoid drinking any aereated drink with your food.

*Tip: If you are scoring most of your iron through plant-based, non-heme sources then get smart about it.*

- *Spinach is loaded with iron, so pair it with orange juice in a green smoothie to absorb the iron better. It is better to have cooked spinach rather than raw as the latter contains oxalates which block the absorption of iron.*
- *Beans and lentils, such as chickpeas/garbanzo beans, white beans, red kidney beans, soybeans, black beans and others, are excellent sources of iron. Prepare them with tomatoes to get maximum benefit.*
- *If you're adding a baked potato as a side, keep the skin on—that's where most of the iron resides.*
- *Tofu; seeds such as pumpkin seeds, sunflower seeds; dried fruits like raisins, apricots; and nuts such as cashews, almonds, pistachio are other good sources of iron.*

**Fun Fact:** Blood donation causes a temporary drop in haemoglobin, but your body makes new red blood cells to replace those that are lost. It's a good idea to eat iron-rich foods for a few days after blood donation.

## 21

# The Important Adaptogens

daptogens are stress-fighting super herbs. Some herbs have superpowers that can help the body adapt to stress and handle it in a healthy way. They strengthen the body and help rebuild our immunity. These wonders are called adaptogens. Adaptogens help to modify the body's reaction to both environmental and internal stress, which, as we all know, is a huge immunity dampener.

## The Popular Ashwagandha

Ashwagandha is actually right up there in the adaptogens list. The anxiety, frustration and mood swings that stress brings in its wake can be debilitating. Ashwagandha is known to help the body adapt to stress by normalizing the levels of cortisol—the stress hormone.

### Know the Adaptogen

This super herb is ancient and its use in medicine dates back three millennia, to the time when the Ayurvedic practitioners in India began using it to help people battling with anxiety and low energy. We now know that this benefit is because of the herb's ability to raise the levels of gamma-aminobutyric acid (GABA), a calming neurotransmitter in the brain.

It is helpful for weight loss in people with chronic stress. It helps boost muscle strength, improves heart and lung capacity to increase energy level, and enhances memory and cognitive functioning. Since it is rich in iron, it also contributes to increased red blood cell count, which is great for those suffering from excessive fatigue. Plus, it works to stabilize blood sugar levels—reducing blood sugar when it's too high or increasing it if too low.

But that's not all. The multiple natural antioxidants and flavonoids in it also help treat inflammation, protect against infection and illness, boost the immune system and promote overall wellness.

## The Immunity Connection

Now it is increasingly getting clear that for those with an underperforming immune system, including ashwagandha in the diet can prove to be a game-changer. It works on multiple fronts. It helps:

- protect against cellular damage caused by free radicals
- increase the production of antibodies in the body, which engulf and digest the toxins and eliminate them from the body
- lower inflammation in the body. This improves the efficiency of the natural killer cells of the immune system, which play a critical role in busting tumours and viral-infected cells
- increase nitric oxide production, which is responsible for activating the immune system's ability to ingest and destroy the toxic invader cells
- enhance the body's immune resistance as it is loaded with flavonoids and multiple antioxidants

## TO-DO

Make ashwagandha tea by boiling ashwagandha powder along with water, milk and tea leaves.

**Fun Fact:** The word ashwagandha is derived from the Sanskrit words *ashwa (horse) and gandha* (smell), alluding to its aphrodisiac properties.

## Moringa: The Buzzy Adaptogen

Foreign superfoods have serious competition from indigenously grown moringa, made from the leaves of the drumstick tree which has been a part of the Indian traditional diet for thousands of years.

### Know the Adaptogen

Moringa leaves are loaded with significant amounts of vitamin A, B, (folic acid, pyridoxine and riboflavin), C and E, calcium, manganese, magnesium, potassium, phosphorous, zinc and protein.

They provide high levels of antioxidants, help balance the hormones, cleanse the gut, nourish the skin, deliver a high amount of calcium and help boost our digestive powers.

**Good to Know**

Moringa is a potent fatigue buster because of the high concentration of iron and magnesium, alongside vitamin A, which increases the absorption of these minerals. This superfood has been discussed in detail in my book *Fix It with Food* and several recipes have been provided to incorporate into your diet.

*The Immunity Connection*

For starters, moringa is high in protein, which is like the skeleton of the immune system. Our immune system's efficiency and functioning depend on a protein-rich diet. Moringa delivers high amounts of all eight essential amino acids that our body needs, making it one of the very few plant foods that deliver complete protein.

Moringa reduces inflammation by suppressing inflammatory enzymes. Moringa also delivers a compound called quercetin, which helps cut inflammation in the body.

It is a fabulous immunity booster, thanks to its high content of potent immunity nutrients—vitamins E and C and a handful of B vitamin. These vitamins, known as the 'antioxidant vitamins', help fight illness and infection.

Finally, as its oxygen radical absorbance capacity (ORAC) value (the antioxidants count) is really high, it helps protect our body, reduce signs of ageing and prevent diseases by fighting off free radical damage from our environment.

---

TO-DO

- You need a very small amount—about 3 grams of powder or about ¼ cup of fresh leaves per day—to score the benefits of moringa. Add moringa powder to your smoothie or cereal, soups and stews.

- If you have access to the tender leaves, boil them in water and sip throughout the day. You could also churn fresh leaves with water, add some lemon juice and honey and enjoy it as a refreshing cooler. Fresh moringa leaves can also be cooked like spinach and other saag.

**Fun Fact:** Moringa, known as a 'never die' plant, is easy to grow, survives in harsh conditions like drought and is good for the environment too.

## Adopt the Humble Amla

Sometimes all we need to do is to look in our backyard to find the superfood we need to score health and combat modern lifestyle diseases. Amla (Indian gooseberry) is a humble, inexpensive, easily available adaptogen. It is India's traditional superfruit.

### Know the Adaptogen

Ayurveda has been advocating amla for a host of health benefits from digestive health to easing cough for ages now. Thankfully, modern science is now recognizing it too.

Amla has a lot going for it. It is 80 per cent water, delivers multiple minerals and vitamins, and has exceptional antioxidant content. Besides being a mild laxative and a diuretic, it is also an effective tonic that restores the appetite, cleanses the liver and is a potent memory booster.

It also protects our cells against radiation and heavy metals and delivers lots of phosphorous, which is needed for proper functioning of the neurotransmitters in the brain and maintaining the health of our bones and teeth.

It is also rich in pectin, which aids in blood sugar control, boosts iron absorption and helps improve acid reflux.

Also, amla has a cooling effect on our body and helps regulate body temperature.

## The Immunity Connection

It is a versatile and powerful antioxidant and due to its antibacterial and astringent properties, it helps fight against various infections, thus, making the immune system strong.

Amla is one of the richest natural sources of vitamin C, a powerful antioxidant that helps protect against various infections and keeps the immune system buzzing.

Amla is also rich in both tannins and polyphenols, both of which make great free radical scavengers.

**Good to Know**

Amla is a rare five-taste herb as it contains five
(all except salty) of the six tastes, or rasas, described
by Ayurveda: sweet, salty, sour,
pungent, bitter and astringent.

---

## TO-DO

- Set a target of eating an amla daily.
- Try having amla and carrot juice as this makes for a powerful duo; carrots deliver loads of beta carotene, which gets converted into vitamin A in the body—a powerful phytonutrient that boosts production of infection-fighting natural killer cells and T-cells. The combination of vitamin A and C makes it a win-win!
- Grate the berry and add to sabzi and salads, or just eat

one every day. If you find it too sour, then boil it with a little salt and turmeric and then eat the fruit.

- Grind amla pieces and strain the juice. Add jaggery, cumin and pepper powder and mix well.
- Cook buttermilk with amla and cumin and pepper powder. When the buttermilk is reduced to half, add salt to taste.
- Amla pickle and amla juice are also very popular, so is amla murabba with those who prefer it sweet.

**Fun Fact:** An amla tree can bear fruits for 65–70 years.

---

## The Holiest of Basil

Do you have a tulsi (holy basil) plant in your house? I bet you do.

Traditionally, tulsi used to be planted in the centre of the courtyard of Hindu houses and was considered an important part of all the religious rituals. It is also thought to release positive spiritual energy and ward off negativity from the house. The health and medicinal benefits of holy basil are well known too.

In fact, holy basil is a herb which is celebrated in the earliest Ayurvedic texts as rasayana, or tonic, that promotes longevity and vitality.

### Know the Adaptogen

Called the queen of herbs, holy basil or tulsi is said to promote purity and lightness in the body and has been used for more than 3,000 years as an antioxidant, antiviral, carminative (gas reliever), diuretic, expectorant, stamina builder, digestive herb, memory booster and is also considered for solving issues related to the nervous system.

It is a powerful adaptogen and is known to encourage tranquillity and clarity, give relief from stress, and function as an effective mood lifter.

## The Immunity Connection

Now, it is increasingly getting clear that tulsi not only works as a caretaker of the body, but it also supports, rejuvenates and strengthens our immunity actively. Regular consumption leads to an increase in cytokines. It also increases the activity of T-cells and natural killer cells, thus boosting the immune system.

Tulsi helps regulate the stress hormone, cortisol levels, which has a direct impact on the immune system.

It contains unique antioxidants and micronutrients that provide powerful immune protection from free radical damage and increase the body's capacity to fight against disease and infections.

**Good to Know**
Tulsi's immune-stimulating properties
make it helpful for fighting environmental allergies.

---

### TO-DO

Tulsi finds its way in many natural remedies that mothers and grandmothers swear by.

- Add it to your tea. Boil the leaves with water, let it brew for a few minutes and finish off with honey and lime juice.

- Have tulsi-infused ghee or honey. Mix powdered tulsi with a spoonful of ghee or honey.
- Drink tulsi juice. To make the juice, blend ½ cup water and 1 cup fresh tulsi leaves to a fine paste. Strain using a fine-mesh strainer and sip it.
- A decoction of tulsi leaves, honey and ginger or tulsi, lemongrass, ginger and jaggery is good for cold, cough, sore throat.

*Tip: Do not chew tulsi leaves as they contain a high amount of mercury and iron which are released on chewing and may cause discolouration of the teeth. You can swallow the leaves or add to a beverage but do not chew them.*

**Fun Fact**: Holy basil is a member of the mint family.

# 22

# The Important Mesonutrients

Remember how grandpa used to insist on eating some raw onion with every meal? And how grandma always insisted on biting into the apple with its peel on? Read on to know why I am reminding you of these.

The nutrition news we are fed is often incomplete, frivolous, half-baked and barely skin deep. However, the truth is, how beneficial certain foods are for us usually lies buried deep within, in some specific components that constitute them.

So, to really understand how to eat well, it's important to go beyond the superfluous information floating around, get acquainted with the good food elements and learn how to score enough of the goodness. Basically, it's time to get acquainted with the mesonutrients, the active compounds found in food that are responsible for some of the amazing health benefits that our favourite superfoods deliver.

## Quercetin: Tiny But Potent

Our health depends not just on food macros. To a huge extent, it depends on the mesonutrients that we miss out on far too often. The first mesonutrient to make friends with is quercetin.

## Know the Mesonutrient

Quercetin is a flavonoid found naturally in many plants and foods like apples, grapes, broccoli and many more. It delivers longer life, relief from allergies, lowered risk of respiratory, skin and GI infections, healthier heart, enhanced energy and more such benefits that all of us seek.

## The Immunity Connection

Quercetin is an anti-cancer, anti-tumour, anti-inflammatory, heart health booster, which improves immunity by fighting free radical damage to help arrest the effects of stress-induced ageing and inflammation.

**Good to Know**

Quercetin is a delicate heat-labile nutrient and may not survive when subjected to boiling water. So instead of boiling tea leaves, place them in a cup, add hot water (not boiling water) and drink as quickly as possible when the brew is ready. That's probably why the Japanese do not boil tea leaves.

---

### TO-DO

- Even though there is no set recommended dietary allowance (RDA) for this antioxidant, we can and must try to get in as much as we can. This is possible by consciously incorporating quercetin-rich foods into our diet.
- For that to happen, we need to know which foods to target: tea leaves, both green and black, are the richest source of quercetin. So a couple of cups a day of both or either is certainly a good idea.

- Other liquids that deliver this mesonutrient are cocoa, cranberry juice, lemon juice (all three are potent sources) and red wine (yes, a little bit of this tipple is good for us).
- Raw red onions are a safe bet too. The white, sweeter variety will give you far less quercetin. So, plate more of the red ones.

### Good to Know

Peel the onions lightly, as most antioxidants are concentrated near the peel. Also, as the quercetin content slightly decreases by cooking, raw is your best bet.

- Next, we have the greens—kale and spinach, and the ubiquitous apple (again the peel has a lot of quercetin). Other foods to score are prunes, peppers, red grapes, dark cherries and berries, tomatoes, broccoli, asparagus, cabbage, sprouts and citrus fruits.
- Also, add some buckwheat to your diet, as this seems to be the only grain with a decent amount of quercetin. Those who designed the Navratri fasting fare, which is usually heavy on buckwheat (kotu atta), really knew their stuff!
- Another interesting (though not so readily available food) loaded with quercetin is bee pollen.

### Good to Know

Quercetin is best when combined with other nutrients such as bromelain or vitamin C because it is not that easily absorbed in the body. Vitamin C and bromelain help to improve its absorption and potency.

> **Fun Fact:** Lovage leaves, a herb similar to parsley and capers, are immature flower buds native to the Mediterranean region. They are the best sources of quercetin.

## Curcumin: A Spice Rack Staple

Today, turmeric is the most feted spice worldwide because of the essential compound—curcumin. This compound, a mesonutrient, found only in this yellow wonder, has made it an international cure—a panacea—and helped indigenous haldi doodh become popular as turmeric latte the world over.

The rising awareness about the mesonutrients depicts that we are now looking for ways to function optimally by exploring the hence unexplored nutrition avenues and focusing more minutely on the idea of plants as medicine.

Curcumin is one such mesonutrient whose rise in the last decade to the status of super stardom has been meteoritic. And thanks to that, turmeric, the spice that delivers this component is considered the gold standard compound in nutrition today.

### Know the Mesonutrient

Curcumin works on all fronts. It slays inflammation, heals the mind, relieves congestion, cleans the blood, strengthens immunity and even boosts our happiness. In a nutshell, it can heal our mind, body and soul.

### The Immunity Connection

Curcumin has strong antiviral properties and reduces the replication of the virus, thus helping in reduction of the viral load.

Though an important part of the immune system to fight infections, when inflammation becomes chronic, it leads to various health problems. Turmeric has shown anti-inflammatory properties that could prevent chronic inflammation. Curcumin is known to suppress various inflammatory molecules which are responsible for the damage caused by viruses.

Curcumin also induces autophagy—the process that helps self-destruct old, useless immunity cells and paves the way to create healthier cells in their place. It is known to target cancer cells while sparing healthy cells. It activates pathways that cause cancer cells to die prematurely. It also blocks pathways that enable these cells to grow, divide and multiply. It helps block enzymes that can cause arthritis inflammation.

---

### TO-DO

- Curcumin is the protector of our protectors—the immune cells in the body—and that's why one of the best ways to boost its count is by having haldi doodh. This way, the benefits double. Milk provides whey protein, which delivers cysteine that helps boost glutathione levels—a master antioxidant that is an unsung miracle immunity booster—and turmeric delivers the miracle compound curcumin that boosts the activity of glutathione enzymes. To make haldi doodh, just warm up some milk, add some pure powdered haldi along with a pinch of pepper. Or just boil some milk with shavings of raw turmeric root, sprinkle some pepper and drink at night before going to sleep. Your body will restore and cleanse as you sleep. Milk will help you sleep better and thus boost your immunity. Curcumin in turmeric is not just anti-viral and anti-inflammatory, it is also immunity-boosting and calming.

- You can use turmeric for tempering your dals and curries liberally; since curcumin is fat-soluble, this is a great way to ingest some of this superfood. Or add a piece of raw turmeric to water, boil it with one teaspoon of ghee and have it every morning. It helps improve immunity and cure dry cough.

## Max Out Its Benefits

- Source pure turmeric to ensure high curcumin level and avoid adulteration or impurities like lead, etc.
- Always pair turmeric with black pepper as the latter contains piperine, which enhances the absorption of curcumin. Somehow our ancestors had cracked this knowledge as most of our traditional recipes have both turmeric and black pepper added in combination.

---

## Glutathione: The Master Antioxidant

If you, like me, can eat spinach every day when in season, or love to add raw tomatoes to every sandwich, or are an ardent lover of guacamole, then you're probably already scoring enough of the lesser-known mesonutrient called glutathione.

It may be an unfamiliar name to you, but glutathione is imperative for our immune system's health. It sits at the centre of the antioxidant defence system in the body and not just affects but actually dictates how our immunity functions. This is not an exaggeration—this antioxidant is *that* important. Yet, it is under-recognized and under-appreciated.

So it's a good idea to become friends with glutathione, a master antioxidant that helps the immune system stay strong and ready to fight infections.

## Know the Mesonutrient

Glutathione is a protein made up of three amino acids—cysteine, glycine and glutamic acid—and is the most abundant antioxidant in our bodies. In fact, virtually every cell in our body has some glutathione in it. Its main job is to protect us. In fact, without adequate levels of glutathione, we can be at risk of multiple medical conditions like stroke, Alzheimer's disease, infertility, chronic obstructive pulmonary disease (COPD), heart disease and more, and optimum levels lead to not just a healthy, disease-free body but also deliver amazing energy, glowing skin, a strong heart, a sharp brain and, of course, a stronger immunity.

It is critical for the detoxification of our body. All the toxins stick onto glutathione, which then carries them into the bile and the stool and out of the body. When glutathione becomes depleted, we can no longer protect ourselves against free radicals, infections, or cancer and we can't get rid of toxins.

## The Immunity Connection

Its effect on our immune system is very definitive.

- It instructs and influences our WBCs to control the inflammation in the body.
- It protects the immune cells.
- It plays a central role in the proper function of T-cell lymphocytes, the mainstay of our immune system, by increasing their numbers.
- It stimulates the production and activity of natural killer cells, our body's front-line infection fighters, to produce more infection-fighting substances to keep both bacterial and viral infections away.

Basically, it is the protector and enabler of our protecting (immune) cells. Look at it like this. When you cut fruit, sometimes you sprinkle some lemon juice on it to keep it from going black, don't you? Antioxidant glutathione works like lemon juice in our body. It counteracts and neutralizes the toxins (free radicals) in the body as soon as they are formed, thus minimizing the damage to the cells and our body, and also detoxes the body naturally.

Secondly, it is excellent at fighting chronic inflammation when inflammation in the body is the root of most new-age disorders that we succumb to these days.

Thirdly, it helps amplify the benefit of vitamin D. When glutathione levels in the body are low, vitamin D cannot work efficiently either. And the connection of vitamin D with immunity is clear. In fact, you need to ensure you have adequate glutathione levels to make sure that your vitamin D3 is working as it should.

Finally, it also boosts (recycles) other immunity-boosting antioxidants, like vitamin C and vitamin E, as well as alpha-lipoic acid and coenzyme Q10 (CoQ10).

### What Leads to Its Deficiency?

Age is the most natural reducer of glutathione levels. As we age, the levels drop naturally, possibly because our body can't create as much.

**Good to Know**
Lower glutathione levels often play a role
in many conditions that are more likely
to develop in older people.

Age is just one factor. There are a number of environmental factors and medical conditions too that can increase the risk of deficiency. These are exposure to pollution, cadmium, UV rays, chronic stress, smoking, excessive alcohol consumption, frequent infections and a poor diet that is lacking in important nutrients.

---

## TO-DO

Glutathione is produced in our body by the liver as a result of a normal function, but sometimes it is not enough. In such a case, a little help through right foods can go a long way to boost their production.

There are a handful of foods that naturally contain glutathione or glutathione-boosting nutrients. It helps to focus on these nutrients and foods.

- Rich dietary sources of glutathione are grapefruits, raw tomatoes, avocados, spinach, asparagus and okra.
- Sulfur from food also helps boost the production of glutathione in the body. It is primarily found in fish and poultry; some vegetarian sources like garlic, onions, chives, asparagus, avocados, spinach and leeks also deliver sulfur.
- Cruciferous vegetables like broccoli, cabbage, cauliflower, radish, arugula, kale are packed with glucosinolates that increase the body's glutathione levels.
- Organ meats, peas, tomatoes, spinach are also good sources as they have alpha-lipoic acid that regenerates and increases levels of glutathione within the body.
- Seafood, eggs, mushrooms, asparagus and whole grains deliver selenium, a trace mineral, which is key in

glutathione production. This mineral is a glutathione cofactor, meaning it is needed for glutathione activity.

- Egg yolk, poultry, yoghurt, red pepper, oats, walnuts and dairy, particularly whey, deliver cysteine which helps boost glutathione levels.
- Vitamin C-rich foods like amla, peppers, kiwi, etc., may help increase glutathione levels by attacking free radicals first, thereby sparing glutathione.
- Vitamin E also helps boost the production of glutathione in the body. Nuts like almonds and peanuts, sunflower seeds, green leafy vegetables like spinach, wheat germ, avocado deliver vitamin E.
- Finally, curcumin found in turmeric assists in restoring adequate levels of glutathione and improving the activity of glutathione enzymes.

## There's More

Chronic lack of sleep may decrease glutathione levels. So focus on scoring enough restorative sleep every day.

Right exercise helps. Completing a combination of both cardio and circuit weight training increases glutathione the most.

*Tip: Excessive exercise without adequate nutrition can actually decrease the levels.*

**Fun Fact:** Glutathione's role as a skin whitening agent is being studied.

## Allicin and Sulphides: The Immunity Superstars

Popping a couple of garlic pods early in the morning may not sound like a palatable prescription, but it works wonderfully because garlic is a triple-bonus food: it's antibacterial, antiviral and anti-fungal. It is our immunity's friend too, thanks to two compounds—allicin and sulphides it is packed with.

### Know the Mesonutrients

Allicin is an oily, slightly-yellow liquid that gives garlic its distinctive odour, helps ease inflammation and block free radicals which harm cells and tissues in the body. Sulphides are oil-soluble organosulfur compounds found in garlic and are known for their curative properties.

### The Immunity Connection

Allicin is a powerful immunity booster that helps the infection-fighting white cells multiply faster, besides increasing the efficiency of antibody production in the body. It also stimulates the activity of natural killer cells, a key element of the immune system that destroys free radicals and viral-infected cells.

Also, garlic has more than 100 sulfuric compounds that are powerful enough to wipe out bacteria and infection. Sulfur compounds that give garlic its pungent smell even assist the body with zinc absorption, which is an important immunity-boosting nutrient. That is why it is a good idea to always add some garlic when cooking high zinc foods like chickpeas and avocado.

**Good to Know**

Sulfuric compounds are also found in brussels sprouts, cabbage, chives, kale, leeks, onions and shallots.

*The Nutrition Punch*

In addition, garlic is an excellent source of manganese and vitamin B6; a great source of vitamin C and copper; a good source of selenium, phosphorus, vitamin B1 and calcium. All these nutrients make it a bonafide immunity-boosting superfood.

---

## TO-DO

Garlic's antimicrobial properties are strongest when it's raw as heat and water inactivate sulfur enzymes, which can diminish its antibiotic effects.

- Crush a few raw garlic cloves and let them sit for a few minutes before gulping it with water first thing in the morning. This helps release the enzymes that are converted into allicin.
- Find eating raw garlic difficult? Place a clove of garlic, sliced very thin between two apple slices and eat. Or chop it small enough to swallow it like a tablet with water. Your breath is not affected, and the garlic still does its thing.
- Cut the garlic. Let it soak in water for 10 minutes and then add hot water, lemon and honey and sip the concoction as tea.
- Chop or mash garlic into a paste (a little salt helps). Let it sit for a few minutes, then spread on a buttered toast. The butter helps soften the bite of the garlic.
- You can also find raw garlic in powder, oil, extract and tablet forms.
- Make it a habit to sauté some garlic in every dish you cook.

- Add some fresh garlic to your pasta sauce or your stir fry.

*Tip: Using more garlic than normal can compensate for the loss of nutrients due to the effects of cooking.*

**Fun Fact:** Garlic contains just four calories per clove.

# 23

# The Essential Nutrient That No One Talks About: Enzymes

There's a lot of information out there about the essential nutrients and their importance in our diet. I know people who are completely oblivious, but I also know many who are encyclopedias on protein, read everything they can on good fats and can list multiple ways to avoid refined carbs in a jiffy.

That said, if you ask me which important constituent of food is the least understood by almost everyone I know—I'd say the enzymes would win hands down.

When I mention enzymes, most people, even those who are fitness enthusiasts and are always updated about the latest superfoods and fad diets, draw a blank. 'They sound familiar...I read about them in school I think...we get them from food, right...' is how I have heard most people describe enzymes. Not many have a clear idea about what they are or what they do.

I feel this is food sacrilege at its worst, simply because enzymes are critical for us, our health and our very existence. Even small amounts of enzymes can make profound changes as they are critical components of every chemical reaction happening in the body. They also help kick-start the very physiological processes that keep us alive and well. They are required for the production of energy, absorption of nutrients, regulation of hormones, healing of wounds, removal of toxins and also for a robust immunity.

That's why it's time for a quick tutorial on enzymes and how they work.

## Know the Enzymes

They came into the limelight when it was discovered that an enzyme found in cows' stomachs could turn milk into cheese. The food industry quickly recognized their importance, and today, enzymes are used in everything from dairy to brewing. But that said, while we have many digestive enzymes naturally present in the body, we still need a regular supply of plant enzymes because chronic stress, illness, pollution, malnutrition and the overuse of medicines can all disrupt our internal synthesis of enzymes.

Also, as most of the food we eat today is way too processed, our diets generally lack in fresh, living, enzyme-rich foods, which creates enzyme deficiencies. This creates havoc in our gut, leading to a medley of uncomfortable gastrointestinal symptoms, including constipation, bloating, cramping and heartburn.

## What Do They Do?

Enzymes are needed to quicken the breakdown of food (carbohydrates, proteins and fats) and also to help absorb these nutrients and get rid of the waste. So, without enough enzymes, food would simply sit in the gut and gradually rot and make our body toxic.

This disruption of the gut balance can also lead to vitamin

and mineral deficiencies as well as a compromised immune system.

Poor absorption of nutrients (due to lack of enough enzymes) can lead to a deficiency of nutritional elements that help the immune function. In fact, as almost 70–80 per cent of the immune system is situated in the digestive tract, keeping up a healthy gut is a significant focal point to help our immunity.

Yes, enzymes are that important, yet there is just not enough dialogue about this important fact.

### Good to Know

To recognize enzyme deficiency, check for frequent allergies, fatigue, bloating, gas, constipation, diarrhoea, indigestion, headaches, mood swings and poor immune function.

## The Immunity Connection

The underlying reason for faulty digestion or a compromised immune system is the lack of enzymes in our diet. For this reason, enzymes should be considered essential nutrients.

In addition, now we also know that enzymes can help slow down the progress of chronic degenerative diseases, dispose of toxins in the bloodstream and cut inflammation from the body. All this helps boost our immunity.

So, it is important to give enzymes the attention they deserve and score enough for the sake of our overall health and iron-clad immunity.

Sadly, our modern diets lack in enzymes in a big way. And as we age, the quantum of enzymes in our body gets depleted further. Get enough enzymes by following these strategies:

- Eating raw foods. Enzymes are ineffective at temperatures above 118°F, so eat some raw food every day. Vegetable juices and salads are an excellent way to ensure that you include raw foods in your diet.
- Eat a wide variety of organic, whole, unprocessed foods to score more enzymes. For example, an apple, high in carbohydrates, contains more amylase than an avocado, which has a high concentration of fat and is high in lipase.
- Cut down on processed foods. Eating enzyme-dead foods burdens the pancreas and other organs, overworks them and eventually exhausts them. And gradually, we lose the ability to digest the food if we continue eating just processed foods.
- Eat sprouts. Nuts, seeds, grains and legumes are very rich in enzymes, but also contain significant amounts of enzyme-inhibitors that prevent enzymes from functioning optimally. So, consume them after soaking, sprouting, fermenting to neutralize the enzyme inhibitors effectively. Sprouting, in fact, actually increases the enzyme content in these foods enormously.
- Get enough magnesium in your diet as this mineral is a coenzyme, which means that it is necessary for the function of enzymes within the body. Green leafy vegetables, fish, seeds, bananas are all good sources.

- Get a regular dose of enzymes from raw, natural products like papayas, figs, pineapples, citrus, berries and raw vegetables like leafy greens, beets, onions, leeks, celery, and herbs like rosemary, fennel and thyme.
- Finally, zero in on foods that promote enzyme production: banana, cucumbers, garlic, onions, coconut, yoghurt, mushrooms and honey.

**Fun Fact:** Wine and beer lovers must know that they get these drinks after fermentation through the action of enzymes.

## Befriend Bromelain

The bottom line is that it pays big time to focus on some tiny, deep-seated food components to ensure that we get and stay strong from the inside. So, it's time to move beyond just the macros like protein, vitamins, etc., and focus on more mesonutrients. Bromelain is one such unsung hero that has been used for centuries by the indigenous people of Central and South America for treating multiple ailments.

### Know the Enzyme

Bromelain is a food component, an anti-inflammatory enzyme found in pineapples. The active ingredients in bromelain include proteinases and proteases, enzymes that break down and digest proteins in the body, that is why it is called a proteolytic enzyme. It also helps our body absorb nutrients more efficiently and thus maximize the benefits of what we eat.

## The Immunity Connection

It helps stimulate a healthy immune system to release inflammation-fighting immune system compounds. This makes it a fabulous immunity booster. It is also one of the most effective natural antihistamines (anti-allergy) and helps keep a lid on respiratory distress and inflammation associated with allergies.

It helps reduce discomfort and swelling associated with sinus problems. So, this compound can be a saviour for those with respiratory issues. Pineapple also helps ease arthritis pain by easing inflammation, besides being a good source of vitamin C, which in turn helps the immune system.

### Good to Know
When bromelain is combined with quercetin, the health benefits delivered by both multiply.

---

### TO-DO

There is only one known food source of this enzyme—pineapple! So, it's a good idea to have some often.

The important thing to remember here is that the fibre-rich core of pineapple has the maximum concentration of bromelain. So, pick the juiciest, ripest one you can find.

### Good to Know
Other sources of proteolytic enzymes are kiwifruit, ginger, asparagus, kimchi, yoghurt and kefir. Papain found in papaya also works along similar lines.

**Fun Fact:** Besides fruit salads and tropical drinks, pineapples are also used to make wine.

---

# IMMUNITY DOWNER

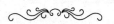

24

# Mind the Sugar Attack

Is it a sprinkle or a shower of sugar for you every day? Do you live on chocolates, rasgullas, cookies and colas? Let's accept it: all of us eat way too much sugar; there is no doubt about that, and we also feel guilty about it.

Now, if you think that only adverse effect of excess sugar consumption is on our teeth and the solution to that is to brush your teeth twice a day, or that sweets are calorific, and we need to 'cut them down' only if we wish to lose weight, then sadly, you are mistaken. Sugar is a far bigger devil for our health than you think.

## The Effects

Excess dietary sugar affects the balance of the body (also called homeostasis,) suppresses the immune system, upsets the body's mineral balance, causes hyperactivity and also adversely affects our immunity.

Unfortunately, most of us don't understand its effect on immunity. And now it's time to change that.

## The Immunity Connection

**The excess weight connection:** Every 5 grams of sugar add an extra 20 calories, and slowly, these calories add up and may lead to weight gain. So if you are skipping meals to lose weight, but not putting a lid on how much sugar you are eating, you are going down the wrong path. Those inches won't melt, and this trail will lead to excess weight, which lowers our immunity too, besides being a direct risk factor for diabetes, heart disease and even liver problems. That's because antibodies that fight infections are not produced effectively if the person is obese—leading to poor immune power in overweight people.

**The inflammation connection:** Excess sugar leads to more inflammation in the body. That is why too many laddoos or chocolates don't show up as just zits on the face (and early wrinkles), or bad skin, but an inflamed body becomes home to multiple adverse health conditions, including a poor immune response.

**The acid connection:** The connection between dental cavities and sugar connection is clear enough, and most of us know that sugar can mess up our 100-watt smile. But that's not all! The truth is that bad bacteria thrive in a sugar and acid environment. More sugar consumption leads to more acid formation, letting bacteria thrive and multiply. This leads to not just more dental issues, but poor overall wellness and immunity too.

**The deficiency connection:** Sugar is a 'quintessential anti-nutrient' that contains no vitamins or minerals (the refinement process of sugar removes all of the sugarcane's natural nutrient). It is 100 per cent carbohydrate, so it must be immediately metabolized. This process devoids our bodies of vital nutrients and negatively affects our immune system.

Digestion of sugar uses the resources already stored in the body. Chromium, zinc, vitamin C, magnesium, calcium, and vitamin B are all needed to digest sugar. This means that eating copious amounts of sugar may actually result in vitamin and mineral deficiencies.

Vitamins B1, B2 and B6 are needed to detoxify and metabolize sugar and can thus be depleted. Sugar also increases magnesium and calcium excretion in the urine and decreases overall magnesium absorption from food.

Excessive sugar consumption can actually deplete the body's nutrient balance that not just upsets the body's mineral balance (making the bones weak), it also often triggers a cascade of inflammation and metabolic disruption. Too much sugar, thus, could lead to severe deficiencies too, which in turn, can lower our immunity.

## That's Not All!

Every time you eat something overly sweet, you temporarily damage the immune system's ability to respond to infections. The effect lasts for several hours (often as much as five hours), so if you eat sweets several times a day—a sweetened cold coffee with breakfast, a can of aerated drinks mid-morning, a sweetened yoghurt for lunch and a cupcake in the evening—your immune system may be operating at a distinct disadvantage all day long.

## Are We Eating Too Much?

Let's accept it, all of us eat way too much sugar; there is no doubt about that at all. Sugar is a hidden toxin that we unwittingly consume at an astoundingly high and unhealthy level. And while there is certainly nothing wrong with having a moderate amount of sugar in your diet, what is damaging is how fast it adds up.

## Good to Know

We should get no more than 10 per cent of our daily calories from added sugar each day. That means we need to limit our sugar intake to no more than six teaspoons, or 25 grams.

---

## TO-DO

- Look out for the umpteen teaspoon of sugar that you add to your tea, coffee, milk, iced tea, lemonade, lassi, cocktails, etc. When it comes to sugar, less is better. Ideally, limit the sugar intake to one teaspoon per cup of coffee or tea, not exceeding two to three cups per day.
- The packaged juices, flavoured yoghurts, canned fruits, cereal bars, chocolates, cookies, aerated drinks (a regular can of cola of 350 millilitres has about 40 grams or 10 teaspoons of sugar), processed foods, granola, sports drinks, even ketchup and salad dressings—all contain added sugar.
- Read labels carefully. Added sugars include all kinds of sugars and syrups put in a product during processing to make it taste better. Look out for raw sugar, glucose, honey, lactose, maltose, molasses, high fructose corn syrup, sorbitol, brown sugar, fructose, fruit juice concentrate or sucrose.
- Keep a check on the carbohydrate content of your diet. To understand, see this simple equation: 4 grams of any carbohydrate breaks down into one teaspoon of sugar in our blood. So, one cup of cooked white pasta is approximately 40 grams of carbohydrate, which breaks down into almost 10 tsp of sugar. If you cut the quantity

to half and add half a cup of vegetables, you will be able to halve the amount of sugar in the meal.

- Stay away from sweeteners. Sweeteners, in fact, can make the problem worse. They may have zero calories, but unfortunately keep the sweet craving and taste alive. So the purpose is not really met.

- It is very important to keep the blood sugar stable by starting the day with a nutritious breakfast and having smaller meals throughout the day to keep sugar cravings away.

- Get 'dessert smart'. It is better to eat sweets in small measures forever than in big greedy quantities and then repent big time. So learn to practice portion control.

- Finally, I don't believe that we need to curb our sugar craving completely and put a blanket ban on all that is sweet. Excess sugar can indeed be bad for us, and if you have diabetes or any other medical condition, you need to go easy on it, but a blanket ban is not needed for the rest of us. I believe that a better strategy is to practice moderation instead of going cold turkey. The fact is that the more you try to run away from sugar, the more you'll think about it and crave it. So, learn instead to get smart about it; choose them right and eat them in moderation.

*Tip: Understand that the first bite gives you the taste of the dessert, the second satisfies you and the third seals the deal. Stop here as any more is simply greed.*

**Fun Fact:** Sugar may give you wrinkles via a process called glycation, in which excess blood sugar binds to collagen in the skin, making it less elastic.

## FACTS TO KNOW 4

### FACTS, ON A LIGHTER NOTE

*Germs can keep us sociable. Yes, our social behaviour is linked to our immune system and our exposure to pathogens.*

*No, you can't eat something that's fallen onto the floor even if you pick it up within five seconds. This five-second rule is a myth since bacteria can instantly hitch a ride on your food.*

# IV

## TAP YOUR MIND

# IMMUNITY BOOSTERS

25

# Cook Mindfully

One exercise I do with everyone is to make them look carefully at their plates and really look at what they are eating. And then take it a step further and analyse how the food reaching their plates is being cooked. This simple task yields a huge payback, always, when done mindfully.

So, what does it yield?

Well, we all eat the same things broadly—potatoes, oranges, carrots, salmon, chicken, rice, eggplant, bread, in varying proportions, of course. But do we all manage the same kind of nutrients and goodness out of the same set of ingredients? Maybe not! Some people manage to derive more goodness from their food and the reasons are actually quite simple.

So, is the potato on their plate healthier than yours?

It is quite possible because how we cook and eat the foods impacts the amount of goodness we derive from them. I have lately been quite obsessed about 'maxing' nutrition from what we eat.

This is my brand of conservation: maximizing the quality and not just quantity because I believe that both processes deliver sustainability and we often fall short on the quality front.

Here are three main ways that can help us do that. You must go through them and see which of these you are following already and which you'd like to begin practising.

## Try To Keep Your Palate Happy

When you eat tasteless or unappealing food (we eat with our eyes too), then the nutrients absorbed from the food are less. Basically, our digestive system gets revved up when we begin to eat something that our brain anticipates enjoying, and the nutrients thus get better absorbed. This means that you'll absorb more antioxidants from a pretty-looking, colourful fruit salad than an insipid, limp, boiled cabbage dish. So, pay attention to aesthetics too as far as food is concerned.

## Zero In on Colour

It is important to know that a diet that is very rich in fruits and vegetables is our best-known bet for preventing almost all chronic diseases. By 'very rich,' I mean simply following the five-a-day rule and making it varied and adding as many different colours of foods as possible.

It is not a tall order, but it still doesn't get done because we are always way too busy or simply uninterested in incorporating them enough into our diet. But it's time to change that.

Science has moved way beyond the macronutrients, protein, fats and carbohydrates. Now it is well known that it is the cocktail of ingredients, the phytochemicals and antioxidants found in fruits and vegetables, which call the shot as far as our health is concerned. These are the ones that repair, energize and help ward off unwanted invaders in the body. Also, try to span the entire spectrum, as the broader the range of colours you eat, the greater the health benefits you reap.

**Good to Know**

It is important not to discard the peels as many (most)
of these phytochemicals are concentrated right there.
Discarding the peel means shortchanging
the nutrients derived from the food and
you wouldn't want that, would you?

## Cook Right

When we cook, it is important not to chop the vegetables into
tiny pieces. In fact, having them as near 'whole' as possible
is a great idea. A simple case in point: potatoes retain 50 per
cent more potassium when cooked whole than when they are
chopped. Similarly, cooked whole carrots retain 25 per cent
more of the cancer-fighting compounds. It is the same for
other vegetables too.

Another critical thing to do is to not leave the vegetables
in water for too long after cutting as most of the electrolytes
leach out. Ideally, wash, then chop and cook right away.

Incorporate these simple changes as we need all the
nutrition we can garner to stay fit in these trying times.

---

### TO-DO

To ensure that you maximize the disease-fighting potential of
foods, here are some of the other steps that you can follow.

- Keep the skin on. You'll be surprised to know that
  potato skin has almost as much protein and even
  more fibre than its flesh. Iron, potassium, magnesium,
  and vitamins B and C are concentrated in the skin. So,
  when you peel it off thickly, you are junking half the
  goodness of the good old potato. This is true for most

other vegetables and fruits. Maximize the potential of apples by keeping their skin on.

- Steam instead of boil. We all know that frying is passé for healthy eaters, but not many know that steaming is a far better way of cooking than boiling to retain nutrients and beneficial plant chemicals like glucosinolates and chlorophyll. It also enhances antioxidant availability. In fact, broccoli cooked in the microwave has been known to lose up to 97 per cent of its antioxidant content; compare this to the 11 per cent loss when it is steamed. And of course, the texture and taste are far better when vegetables are steamed than boiled. Get a good steamer if you find the process cumbersome. It's a super worthwhile investment. And when eating out, look out for dishes that are steamed. Your body will thank you for it.
- Eat more home-cooked meals. Eating home-cooked food ensures that you eat better quality food, and you are also more likely to be aware of what you consume when you prepare it, which will make you less likely to overeat. This one change can make a world of difference to what you eat and your health status as well. That's because when you cook at home, you have more leeway to choose the ingredients that go into making your food. You have much more control; you can get smart about the food that makes it to your plate and consciously pick what is higher in fibre and lower in salt, sugar and calories. In truth, a healthy diet contains plenty of delicious and satisfying foods. So make this change—cook your own meals, and notice the difference on your wallet and on your health.
- Use the right pots to cook. Getting a little experimental

in the kitchen helps, be it with ingredients, seasonings, or even just the way we cut the veggies. It helps keep boredom away, opens up our palate to different tastes and flavours, and may add more nutrients to the fare we eat. Another great way to do this is to take a second look at the way we cook, and the pots and pans we use. Our ancestors cooked in a fuss-free, uncomplicated, absolutely natural way. Maybe they were on to something. Let's try and incorporate their ways and use more earthen, stainless steel and cast-iron pots.

- Slow down. Please eat mindfully. Take time to chew and enjoy your vegetables. The age-old rule says chew each bite 20 times, but if that is too much for you, then do your best. Remember, the more you chew, the more you will break down vegetables, resulting in better absorption of nutrients in the gut.

**Fun Fact:** The fear of cooking is a recognized phobia and is called mageirocophobia.

# 26

# Breathe Right

Imagine having a tool at your disposal that can help calm your mind within minutes. Well, breathing exercises are that tool which do not just help detoxify the body but also help combat the negative effects of stress on our health and immunity. Let me explain how this works.

When our body perceives a threat from the environment, it releases stress hormones namely, cortisol, epinephrine and norepinephrine, which activate our sympathetic nervous system and leads to an increase in the blood flow in the body, shallow breathing, higher heart rate and insulin levels, shutting down of the digestion and reproductive systems, and nosediving of our immunity.

On the other hand, when we are stress-free, our parasympathetic nervous system is activated where all systems of the body function at an optimum and the immune system is also at its efficient best, ready to take on any infections that attack us. It's a no-brainer thus that we want the parasympathetic nervous system to be more active to stay in good health and stay safe from infections. Thus, our breath is an indicator of our mood and our mood is an indicator of our breath. It means that our breathing pattern changes with our mood. It also means that we can change our mood if we change how we breathe.

So how can we switch on this system and move the

body away from the stress-induced sympathetic system? This can be done by controlling our breath. How we breathe can change the message our body gets. Shallow, short breaths, which we take when we feel threatened, tell the body that it needs to be stressed and release stress hormones, which continue to create havoc, whereas controlled breathing can be a gamechanger and move the body to the rest and repair mode. Long and deep breaths help slow down the heart rate and reduce the threat perception; thus, they help switch on the parasympathetic nervous system.

## How Does Breathing Help?

Two things happen when we take deep, intentional breaths from the belly (as opposed to our chests). Deep breaths activate the vagus nerve in the gut, which is a thick nerve connected to the brain. On activation, it transfers the serotonin produced in the gut to the brain, helping us calm down instantly. That is how slow, deep breathing techniques help activate the parasympathetic nervous (PSNS) system. Secondly, belly breaths also activate the diaphragm—the thin skeletal muscle underneath the heart and lungs that separates them from the abdominal cavity. An active diaphragm works splendidly as a detoxifying agent and helps to throw out excess toxins, stress hormones, etc., from the body.

Correct breathwork cannot just make us more energetic and help clear a lot of mental fog; it also strengthens digestion; as about 70 to 80 per cent of our immune tissue is situated in our digestive tract, correct breathing can improve the body's immune response. This also provides more oxygen to the blood, reduces stress levels and fights anxiety—all help boost the immune system additionally.

Ancient yogis called this way of breathing 'fasting of breath' (akin to the fasting of food) and considered it an essential tool for seeking health and preventing and curing illnesses. They believed that it delivers great power to the mind, body and consciousness, and now science is proving them right. It has now been found that controlled rhythmic breathing and breath-holding can increase natural killer cells. That is why divers (who need to hold their breath for a long time) usually have a higher number of natural killer cells.

## Look Out

These are the five big breathing mistakes we make:

- Only breathing into the chest
- Inhalations are stronger and longer than exhalations
- Mouth breathing
- Reverse breathing (where the diaphragm rises instead of falling on the inhale)
- Over-breathing (rapid and deep breathing which may leave one breathless)

### Good to Know

Most of us tend to be right nostril dominant which means we breathe more through the right nostril. It is believed that this activates the sympathetic nervous system making us more fired up and active. When the left nostril is dominant, we are relaxed and at ease. Single-nostril breathing can help regulate the left and right sides, thereby creating balance in our nervous system.

## Correct Your Posture

Another factor that matters is our posture. Dependence on technology, bad work environments and everyday stresses have ruined our posture, and this impacts our major breathing muscle, the diaphragm. When we sit in the wrong posture, our lungs compress (as the upper back is pushed forward and the neck is craning forward) and we can't breathe optimally. When we breathe wrong, that is, breathe faster due to hunched shoulders and tense muscles, our body takes it as a signal of threat, and activates the 'fight or flight' response. Stress hormones flood our body and the sympathetic nervous system gets activated. Having a bad posture and bad breathing habits will harm your body.

Think of a yoga guru who is really old; what image comes to your mind? Isn't it usually a person with an erect spine and perfect posture? Those who do yoga are very concerned about the correct posture and there is a big reason for that. They believe that our energy chakras are situated in our spine. If the spine is straight, the energy between these chakras flows well, and a bad posture obstructs the flow of energy and vitality and messes with our immunity.

So, correct breathwork can help combat the stressors in our life, lead to enhanced immunity and slow down ageing. So consciously learn to:

- exhale longer
- breathe deep enough to activate your diaphragm
- fix your posture

## How To Breathe Right

The first rule is always to take long, deep and slow breaths that move beyond your chest and go down to the belly. When you breathe in, your stomach should go out and when you breathe out, your stomach should go in. Keep your hand over both the stomach and the chest to see if that is happening.

The second rule is that your exhalation should be longer than your inhalation—exhalation switches on the rest and recover mode.

The third rule is to do deep breathing exercises consciously every day; even five to 10 minutes help.

A few breathing exercises that you can try are:

- Slowly breathe in and count to 10. Breathe out very slowly while counting to 10. The next day, increase your count to 15 and then 20 until you can reach 100 counts. While you practise this breath-control, you will strengthen your lungs. The best time to do this exercise is early in the morning or just before you fall asleep.

- Trapped, stale air inside us is what causes shortness of breath. So, before you can breathe in the fresh air, you need to get the old air out. Try this—first relax, let your neck and shoulders droop. Then breathe in slowly, purse your lips in a whistling position, and blow out slowly and evenly. Try to take at least twice as long to breathe out as you did breathing in. Repeat until you no longer feel breathless. Practise pursed-lip breathing several times each day.

Kavita Devgan

- Stand straight. Be relaxed. Keep your arms at your sides and your feet slightly apart. Take a few deep breaths and exhale through the mouth. But don't stop here, because there is still air left in your lungs. Some air always remains in the lungs and is not replaced with fresh air as we breathe. Now, force your diaphragm to exhale all the air from your lungs with a wheezing sound. Do this several times, exhaling through your mouth with a deep puff until you feel there is no more air in the lungs. At this point, you will notice that you have pulled in your belly towards the spine. Slowly inhale fresh, clean air into your empty lungs through your nose. Fill your lungs with fresh air, and then hold your breath for five seconds, counting them slowly. Repeat the process to expel the remaining air out of the lungs. Repeat as many times as you like but at least 50 times each day.

- Sit upright or cross-legged on a firm surface. Keep your back straight and hold one nostril closed with your finger. Inhale deeply through the other nostril while keeping your mouth closed. Exhale through your mouth and repeat 15 to 20 times with each nostril. This helps to improve nasal breathing, which cleanses and warms the air before it reaches the lungs.

- Stand up straight with your arms at your sides and inhale through your nose in three short breaths, almost as though you are sniffing. While you inhale, lift your arms from your sides to your shoulders and up over your head. Exhale through your mouth while lowering your arms back to your sides. Repeat this exercise 10 to 12 times. This exercise helps open up the lungs to facilitate respiration.

**Fun Fact:** Breathing slowly and taking longer breaths can reduce appetite and help cut food cravings and addictions.

Kavita Devgan

# 27

# Eat Stress-Free

R aise your hand if you eat in the car, in front of the television, or at your work desk often.

Now raise your hands again if you suffer from heartburn, indigestion, nausea, constipation and lowered immunity.

If you eat in situations like those mentioned above, where you are barely looking at the food, then there is no point in focussing on eating healthy, as the stress of the situation (how you eat) will not allow the body to absorb the nutrients well, even if you plate the most amazingly nutritious food every day.

And it's a no-brainer that low nutrition equals low immunity.

## Why Does This Happen?

Focussing on how you eat is as important as what you eat. This is because our digestion actually begins in the brain, not in the mouth and the stomach (as most of us think).

This is how it pans out—the look of the food or its thought triggers saliva production in the mouth and the stomach acid. This ensures that by the time we actually begin eating, the mouth and the salivary enzymes are already primed to break down the food's nutrients.

Also, when we eat 'minus' stress, we focus on the food

more and chew each bite carefully, increasing our ability to absorb maximum goodness from the food. This way, when the food reaches the stomach, the acids waiting there are able to break down the protein, fat, carbs, fibre further, isolate nutrients more effectively, and absorb the minerals, vitamins and antioxidants to the fullest.

The supply of nutrients from the food we eat is what elevates our immunity and lowers our chances of falling sick. So, a lack of these nutrients can be detrimental to our health.

Simply put, when we eat under stress the entire process gets compromised, the brain is caught sleeping, or rather it is busy doing other stuff (like looking at a screen) and the nutrients' absorption thus gets seriously shortchanged.

## In a Snapshot

When we eat without stress, the normal physiology of digestion—saliva, stomach acid and all digestive enzymes—works better. In a fight and flight mode (stress mode), the entire digestion gets compromised—decreased saliva, napping stomach acids, less efficient pancreas and lax bile enzymes. All this contributes to poor absorption of nutrients. Eating in this mode also triggers indigestion and heartburn very often.

## There's More!

Eating under stress inhibits the normal contractions of the intestines too, messing the digestive process further, often leading to chronic constipation—a condition that is a known harbinger of multiple diseases.

## Final Word

Our mindset during meal times affects our digestion. Optimum nutrition (and thus optimal immunity) involves paying attention to what we eat and how we eat it. So, eating mindfully and stress-free can actually be a very effective (and easily practised) immunity booster.

### Good to Know
Poor nutrition can make your stress worse too. A well-nourished person handles a stressful situation better than a poorly nourished one.

---

### TO-DO

- Separate your mealtime from task time, entertainment zone and socializing window.
- Consciously get into the rest and low-stress mode before you begin eating. It helps to take a few deep breaths before your mealtime to calm the frayed nerves.
- Say a prayer, even a short one-line prayer will do, or express gratitude for the food you are about to eat. This simple practice has solid science behind it. It'll help you focus on the task ahead of eating the food and serve as a breakup point from whatever you were doing earlier, however stressful that might be.
- Look at the food and eat. Look at every bite you take in (and not at a screen). Your body absorbs what you see.
- Chew food well and then swallow. This helps turn on all of our senses and gives the stomach time to handle the food coming its way more efficiently.

**Fun Fact:** Eating slowly results in feeling full sooner and thus eating fewer calories at mealtimes.

## 28

# Tap the Mind Energy

Our perception of our bodies is wrong; rather, it is incomplete.

When we talk about our body, we only consider the tangibles—the organs, the systems and we completely discount the energy that goes through our body. Medicine completely ignored this aspect too, until 1925, when quantum physics was discovered, and brought about a change in thinking and how solutions for illnesses are perceived, pursued and found.

Let me put it this way—our body is made up of cells, which are made up of DNA comprising atoms (protons, neutrons and electrons) and inside the atom, there is nothing.

It is mostly empty space between subatomic particles, and it is here that the energy of our body resides.

## What Is This Energy?

Consciousness and invisible energy from the mind shape our body, and now we are aware that it has a lot of power over our psychology and our biology. New thinking now believes strongly in the mind-body connection and a holistic approach that includes our mind, body and emotions to prevent and even treat illnesses is picking up speed.

Thinking, believing and the tone of our emotions all lead

to chemical, biological and physiological changes in the body. The idea gaining huge ground today is that 'belief itself shifts our biology', and that there is an innate capacity of our body to heal. But it only works if you actually first accept, then believe and finally surrender to this idea. Alternate treatments work around this idea. With surrender, the body begins training the autonomic nervous system to make its own healing chemicals and they help treat the condition.

This approach is not a quick-fix application, but that doesn't mean that it doesn't deliver results. In any case, it is becoming increasingly clear that with chronic diseases that develop over a long period of time, quick-fix approaches don't really work anyway.

There is now enough scientific evidence to corroborate that effective remedy involves getting down to the roots and the body's basic energy imbalance. That is why positive thinking is a big tool used by most of the alternative treatments (where the basic belief is that the human body was born to heal and has renewable cells and capacity for emotional healing).

The other side of this coin is negative thinking, which is equally potent as it works in the opposite direction and can be very destructive. While positive thinking (placebo) heals and cures, negative thinking and beliefs (nocebo) can cause illnesses. This field of study is called epigenetics.

## The Immunity Connection

Epigenetics follows a belief that our nervous system systematically sends information about both the external and internal environments of our body to different organs and even to our immune system. Then our mind interprets our environment, the stressors, our perceptions, our thinking and our beliefs—all this plays a huge role in deciding what signals we send to our organs and our immune system.

Positive beliefs = positive and healing signals

Negative beliefs = negativity and debilitating signals

This makes all the difference.

**Good to Know**

Even if we can't change the situation, or the environment, just by changing our perception of the environment (positive or negative), we can influence our genetic activity positively or negatively.

We must remember that there is a mind between our environment and our cells, and its powers are very strong.

## Power of Belief Is Everything

Our belief directs our immune system to be either in fight or flight or in rest and repair mode. The environment in which we live, of which, our thinking and beliefs are a huge part, selects and directs the genetic activity of our cells. People with the same cells and the same genetic susceptibility can behave differently. One can heal and the other deteriorate just because the former has learnt to optimize the genetic activity by controlling the environment and the latter has given up and is dwelling in negativity (nocebo).

## It's Simple

When our heart sends out sorted, coherent and happy signals to our brain, the brain sends out signals that support our immunity. On the contrary, the stress signals (chaotic zagged waves) force the brain to undermine our immunity. This happens because with chaotic stress signals, our body systems—say, the blood or the lymphatic system—does not work effectively; the body then becomes more acidic, leading to inflammation and in turn, lowered immunity.

## In a Nutshell

The healing process involves breaking the bad habits that cause destruction, making new, better choices, overcoming limited thinking, cutting loose debilitating emotions and beliefs, and thus beginning the reverse process towards healing.

---

### TO-DO

- Make a deliberate attempt to stop absorbing negative thoughts, energies and emotions of the people around you. Our subconscious mind is shaped from these influences and, in turn, affect our genetic make-up.
- Trauma around you—alcoholism, toxic relationships, conflict, trauma, drama, uncontrolled tempers, constant complaining—all are processes that not just affect our emotions at that particular time, but they also settle so deeply that we keep feeling them over and over again throughout our life. They affect our biology for a long, long time. It is thus imperative to consciously shake off their effects. And the best way to do this is to accept these influences and then let go of the past consciously and with determination.
- Emotional blockages due to anger, trauma, grief and frustration lead to unpleasant feelings that prevent us

from moving forward and cloud our thought processes. In addition, they lead to physical blockages that may develop into a disease. That is why it is important to diffuse them timely. The release can happen in multiple ways—exercise, conscious breathwork, soul cleansing, meditation, hypnotherapy. Letting go of negative emotions—especially those that we have suppressed and locked away in our brain someplace deep—is crucial and needs to be done consciously,

- Practising forgiveness is akin to self-healing. It is the most effective way of purging negativity and healing, and healing equals immunity. So let go of the victim mindset.

- Practise meditation. It helps shut down the fear response and switches on the parasympathetic nervous system, which switches on the relaxation response and heals. It helps to purge residual negativity from the body. Also, during meditation, the pituitary gland releases oxytocin, dopamine, serotonin, endorphins—chemicals that are all good for us.

  With meditation, cortisol levels decrease and immunoglobulin (IgA) levels (our primary defence against bacteria and virus in our body) increase substantially. That is why practising meditation regularly can help keep us in a state of continuous healing.

  There are a lot of ways to meditate. Transcendental meditation is the form where you repeatedly chant a mantra that competes with your thoughts for your complete and total awareness.

  The idea behind every meditation is to quieten the chatter in mind and slow down breathing. This can happen during any activity, for example, even during a walk.

- Visualize. Use this tool for active healing because what we imagine affects our physiology. Just actively imagining wellness instead of illness can work wonders.
- Loving thoughts, gratitude and appreciation also heal. These lead to the release of oxytocin, which boosts natural killer cells and WBCs in the body, which strengthen our immunity. So, keep those hugs coming.
- Faith healing is not very well understood yet, but it works and it has been seen time and again that faith has the power to interject and change the trajectory of the disease and lead us to miraculous healing and better immunity.

**Fun Fact:** Meditation as a practice is thought to be around 2,600 years old.

# 29

# Become a Cautious Optimist

McLandburgh Wilson, a famous author, wrote in 2015, 'The optimist sees the doughnut, but the pessimist sees the hole.' While doughnuts have never helped anyone's health, how we think—positively or negatively—can definitely affect our health extensively. In fact, optimism is a potent health tonic.

Our body takes its cues from how we are feeling, so a positive outlook adds to our health and a negative outlook is detrimental to it. Practising a glass-half-full attitude actually helps strengthen the immune system immensely. This is precisely why optimists tend to live longer than pessimists.

On the other hand, those who are constantly negative, moody, nervous and easily stressed tend to have a weaker immune system and fall sick more often. That is why if your workday starts off bad, you need to tell yourself and truly believe that it could only get better. And so, if you can't go out to eat and meet with friends due to the pandemic, you need to learn to be genuinely happy that you can use the extra time baking some goodies at home and enjoying them with family. Ruing what is missing can be a potent health downer.

Knowledge is the key to staying healthy, and optimists not only engage in healthier behaviours like sleeping enough, exercising regularly and choosing foods carefully, they also tend to track their health more closely.

**Good to Know**

While optimism appears to protect the heart, being pessimistic, cynical and hostile may lead to higher blood pressure and heart disease risk, among other health issues.

## The Immunity Connection

Immunity is one area where our thoughts and attitudes can have a very powerful influence.

It's got a lot to do with our attitude. Optimists and pessimists approach problems differently and their ability to cope successfully with adversity differs as a result. Pessimistic people tend to view problems as unchangeable and extensive, whereas optimistic people are the opposite. While dealing with a challenge, an optimist will typically believe in confronting a problem head-on and finding ways to reduce its severity and fix the problem. Instead of giving up hope (like pessimists), they would cope with stressful situations far better than a pessimist.

Optimists also manage their relationships better and usually have more friends. So when they face an adverse health event, they have a network to rely on for support, which helps them manage the resulting stress more effectively. All this helps counter the ill effects of stress and protects against the inflammatory damage of stress.

Secondly, when we are optimistic, there is a stronger cell-mediated immunity (CMI), that is, a higher flood of immune cells respond to an invasion by foreign viruses or bacteria. Whereas when we are pessimistic, the CMI is weakened, leading to a sluggish immune response.

Along with it, activation in brain areas associated with

negative emotions leads to a weaker immune response to a flu vaccine.

## The Catch

Optimism can have both positive and negative immune correlations. When stressors are brief and seem manageable, then optimism appears to be protective against their bad effects. But this effect is reversed when stressors are prolonged, that is, they last longer and go out of hand.

So, when circumstances are easy or viable, optimism is good for the immunity because it can lead you to finding a solution and towards closure of the stressor. However, under extremely difficult circumstances, a person should disengage or give up instead of trying unceasingly to optimize a lost situation.

When circumstances are difficult or complex, optimism can negatively relate to immunity because it leads to ongoing engagement with persistent stressors. Cutting corners for a lost case can actually be physiologically protective as it minimizes the exposure to the stressor.

Cautious optimism and keeping expectations realistic, thus, is a perfect way to keep your immune system alive and kicking! And there is no doubt that more positive and and hopeful people tend to live healthier.

---

### TO-DO

- Stop taking the blame for bad news, stop assuming that the situation will last forever and will affect everything you do. In short, stop being a pessimist. Never assume blame for negative events, learn to give yourself credit for good news, believe that good times and things will last and go on to make your life good in all aspects.

- Feeling better about the future might help you feel better for real. So, visualize an ideal future—landing your dream job, living with a loving partner or moving bag and baggage to the country of your choice. Write it all down in a journal entry. Just doing this simple process can help increase the feeling of well-being.
- Count your blessings and feel grateful for them. This is a sure-shot way of getting optimistic about yourself and your situation.
- Practise reframing. For example, when you are stuck in a traffic jam, instead of stressing about it, appreciate the fact that you can spend a few extra minutes listening to music.
- Practise gratitude. Gratitude is associated with optimism, and grateful people are generally happier, less stressed and less depressed.
- The world is full of all kinds of news; consciously focusing on the positive news and disregarding the negative helps to centre yourself in positivity.
- Cultivate healthy emotions like contentment and hope on a daily basis. Focused optimism is linked to a rise in positive emotions, which are associated with sturdier immunity.
- Selectively remembering the positive memories can help boost your immune functioning just when you need it the most.
- Build resilience as that helps in the long run. Resilience is the ability to adapt to stressful and negative situations and losses. And the best news is that resilience can be cultivated by nurturing positive emotions regularly.

Kavita Devgan

- Finally, optimism can be learnt. It can be developed and nurtured, so practise this consciously and mindfully.

**Fun Fact:** Winston Churchill famously said, 'A pessimist sees the difficulty in every opportunity; an optimist sees the opportunity in every difficulty.'

# IMMUNITY DOWNERS

## 30

# Put a Lid on Stress

The kind of stress we face has changed over the centuries. Earlier, when our ancestors faced life-threatening situations, like saving themselves from a wild animal or surviving a natural calamity, the body would react by mobilizing all resources to make survival a reality. Today, the kind of stress we face has changed—that wild animal has taken the shape of an angry boss or a furious spouse, and that natural calamity probably shows up in the form of an empty bank balance and a massive credit card payment that is due soon.

Unfortunately, it is difficult to define stress, as what may appear to be a stressful situation for one person is not so for another. It can come in the form of losing a job, bankruptcy, retirement, demonetization, divorce, personal illness or injury, death of a family member or spouse, the list goes on and on.

However, while the stressors have changed substantially, the way the body physiologically reacts to stress is still the same. There is a fight or flight response that triggers every time we are stressed and it takes away resources and energy from everywhere else in the body—the gut, the brain, the immune system—and gives it to the muscles to ward off the 'perceived' threat.

While this lasts, all organs work at less than optimum—we don't digest the food properly, our memory takes a beating, the toxins don't get thrown out and the body cannot fight against invaders, which obviously undermines the immune system from all sides. This cycle gets repeated every time we face a stressful situation. Over time, too much stress, too often, can shut down our immune system. The connection is as direct as that.

## Not All Stress Is Bad

Short-term and moderate stress, like projects for school or meeting a work deadline, may in fact, be good for us as it makes our brain work in high gear and leave us with a satisfying feeling at the end of the task.

But chronic stress—weeks or months of stress—is not good for your body and immune system. If the stress continues for years, the damage can be severe. This kind of stress, along with the sudden and unpredictable stress (for example, the loss of a loved one) that throws our bodies off, can wreak havoc on our health. That's because the way we think, the emotions that cruise through us, even the quality of our relationships are all invisible influences which result in physical and chemical changes in the body.

## The Hidden Damage

The problem is that we all complain about the symptoms instead of the main issue. Bad moods and temper tantrums, lost appetites and a million lousy spinoffs and side effects in between...that's how stress vexes us. But we never think beyond...and try to figure out what stress could really be doing to us inside.

There really is no escaping the fact that stress affects our health badly. In the beginning, the body's response to stress may be a headache, back strain or stomach pain, or it may zap your energy, wreak havoc on your sleep and make you feel cranky, forgetful and out of control. But if we are constantly stressed, it may lead to a constant hormonal battle that can lead to troubles like hypertension, diabetes, heart disease, inflammatory disorders, lowered immunity, autoimmune disorders and more.

When stress increases, the blood-brain barrier allows chemicals to pass through it, and harmful chemicals and foreign bodies affect the neurons and the brain adversely.

## The Immunity Connection

Have you ever noticed how you come down with a cold or flu when faced with stressful situations like final exams or relationship problems? There is a field of psychology called psychoneuroimmunology that studies how our state of mind affects our state of health. The connection between the mind and body is well established. The phrase 'you are worrying yourself sick' is true!

Chronic stress harms our immune system's efficiency and undermines its ability to mount a response to invading offenders and fight off the antigens, making us sitting ducks for infections.

Stress creates a hormone in our body called cortisol. Cortisol helps the body manage stress by toning down any non-essential operations in the body. Unfortunately, during this process, it also puts on pause the immune functions in an effort to conserve energy, making stressful periods the perfect time for germs to get a toe in and settle down.

When stress lasts longer, like days or weeks, increased cortisol levels can start to have more negative effects. Elevated cortisol suppresses the immune system by reducing the production of WBCs.

Without enough WBCs, the lookout for germs gets inefficient and response to infection becomes much slower. That is why long periods of cortisol elevation can leave us susceptible to illnesses we otherwise could have easily dodged.

Now you know why you come down with a fever after a long stint of stressful exams or a project deadline that was too tight.

## The Inflammation Connection

In addition, when there is too much cortisol in the blood for a long time, it spikes up inflammation, which is bad news for our immunity. When we are chronically stressed, cortisol output is first increased and ultimately reduced. When levels are too low—caused by a resistance to cortisol created due to chronically high levels over time—we become desensitized to cortisol over time, losing the ability to fight inflammation adequately. This leads to increase of inflammation in the body.

High-stress levels can cause depression and anxiety, which add to inflammation. Sustained high levels of inflammation are actually an indication that the immune system is overworked and over-tired and cannot protect us properly.

To compound things, when our bodies have elevated stress levels, the nervous system begins to accept this heightened stress level as normal and continues to produce high levels of stress hormones long after the stressful event has passed, further compromising the immune system.

Stress very often affects behaviours that are known to down our immunity: smoking, drinking, loss of sleep, physical inactivity and overeating—eating too much sugar and processed foods. So if stress makes people resort to drinking too much alcohol or smoking more, or snack on junk food, these habits also directly impact our immunity and compromise it.

Stress really does attack our immune systems in multiple, deadly ways and is highly debilitating for our system.

### Good to Know

When a woman undergoes a lot of psychological stress during pregnancy, the developing infant's brain can get affected by the surge of neurochemicals and hormones in the mother's body. This, in turn, can weaken and impair the infant's immune system tremendously.

---

### TO-DO

Learning to manage the stress in your life can help keep cortisol levels down and protect your immune system. Try these sure-shot stress busters to prime your body.

- **Exercise**: The endorphins released boost your efficiency, perk up your spirit and dissipate stress. A sweating session also promotes the production of neurohormones in the brain that are associated with improved cognitive function and elevated mood. Even better news is that this positive mood endures for a few hours. In addition, exercise reduces anxiety and equips us to react better when confronted with emotional events.

  So tie up your laces and go out for a run now (and every day). Are you pressed for time? Weave it in your work life. Go for a 20-minute walk around the block during lunch hour, sneak to the office (or nearby) gym in the afternoon hours when work is slack, and every three hours or so, stand up and stretch your muscles. Even cycling is great as its rhythmic flow (repeat action) can relax your mind completely!

- **Meditate**: For long-term stress relief, believe in the power of meditation. It can help manage anxiety, depression and pain. You don't really have to follow a school of meditation; just sit quietly for 20–30 minutes in the early morning to start the day well. This is also the time when you can focus your energies on doing things well and set yourself in the right mode for the day ahead.

- **Carve out some downtime**: Do this consciously— for example, press pause when you are having lunch. Don't entertain anyone, anything during this time— no calls, no discussions, no arguments. Take a total break from everything. Ideally, even put your phone on silent. Similarly, zero in on the half an hour or so after you wrap up work for the day to relax and unwind.

- **Choose carefully**: Relationships and people can be big stressors. Try not to be around people who leave you wondering/tired/angry/frustrated. So instead of tricky confused people, be with honest, straightforward people and there'll be a lot less stress. It is easier said than done, but give it an honest shot and you'll be surprised with the benefits.

- **Learn time management**: Most people feel stressed because they have little time or energy for themselves and for the things that matter to them. For starters, take an honest look at your schedule, get more realistic and drown out expectations from others. Invest in a session or two with life and time-management coaches who can train you to organize your life better, identify the pressure points and help you make constructive changes that can reduce stress.

- **Cut the clutter (in your home, your work cubicle, your car and so on):** Clutter directly adds to stress in your life. It's not as popular a resolution as vowing to drop weight but shedding unwanted stuff and getting organized is equally essential for your health and sanity (and immunity). Changing your physical environment goes a long way towards changing your state of mind. When you declutter, you get back in control and free yourself. Besides, letting go of useless material delivers potent mental upliftment too.

- **Get out:** Spend 30 minutes outdoors every day. Sunlight is every bit as essential to our well-being as proper nutrition and exercise. That's because our bodies make vitamin D when our skin is exposed to sunlight, and vitamin D, responsible for neuronal growth, has a positive effect on our mood. Secondly, the brain produces more of the mood-lifting chemical serotonin on sunny days than darker days. Exposure to sunlight also stimulates the pineal gland to produce melatonin which plays a role in proper sleep (again, an effective de-stressor).

Here are a few quick-fix solutions that you can easily add to your lifestyle.

- **Switch to green tea:** A substance in green tea leaves, l-theanine, can shift brain wave activity from the beta waves that accompany anxiety to the alpha waves associated with relaxation.

- **Stretch in the shower:** The hot water will loosen up your muscles, so it's easier to get a good stretch. The act of stretching will help to release stored tension and help you begin the day feeling more relaxed, at peace and ready to handle what comes your way. You can end the day the same way too.

- **Just escape:** Endless e-mails, voice messages and friends and coworkers all vying for your time and attention? Work and life can both be super stressful. Simply close your eyes. Picture yourself stretched out on a white, sandy beach with an endless blue sky above, listening to waves crashing at your feet. After this little 'you time', you'll come out ready and equipped to handle the world. When things get just too much to handle, simply step into your room and stay there. Let your mind go on a holiday. Take a good book and just lie back and read, or listen to music; shut the world out.

- **Change your attitude:** A delay stresses most people—it could be a hold-up in achieving a goal, not reaching a place on time or something similar, but instead of fretting, take a deep breath and tell yourself that in the bigger scheme of things, something not happening on time today is really unimportant. Similarly, even when the worst happens at work, a big deal collapses or targets are seriously unachievable, you still have two choices: sulk in a corner and tremble maybe or try thinking about what the situation will look like a year or two from now. Will it still be so earth-shatteringly important? Look at everything from that perspective. Accepting is often a key factor in handling stress. Also, stop worrying about the things you have no control over and concentrate only on what you have the power to change.

- **Break the monotony**: When was the last time you tried something new—something that seemed strange and not very comfortable? Go on, do it now. Not only will it make life more interesting, it'll also keep your brain buzzing and keep your soul in good shape. Explore new cuisines. You will find new ingredients and your taste buds will tingle with newness. Maybe go to a beach on your next vacation, instead of heading to the hills yet again, or try reading non-fiction (give your brain something different to chew on), or take lessons in shooting or salsa.

- **Bank on humour**: It portrays spunk and hope and can really help ease stress. Who doesn't want a bit of cheering at any and every given point in life? You can keep a collection of jokes and cartoons and at least one humour book on the desk; you can turn coffee breaks into humour breaks. Take 10 to 15 minutes, particularly during the most stressful parts of your day, to share something funny with a friend or colleague. When you feel stressed, take a moment and read something funny and laugh out loud.

- **Cuddle up now**: It's not just children who need hugs. Adults benefit from them too. Holding hands and hugging can measurably reduce stress and that's because hugs send calming messages to the brain and slow the release of cortisol.

- **Go on a 'sniffari'**: Aromatherapy was once considered new age and kooky. These days it is often used to relieve stress. Chamomile, lavender, melissa, lemon balm or frankincense are the essential oils that help calm the nerves and mind both.

**Fun Fact:** Stress is one of the greatest 'stealers' of productive time and it is the number one reason for people to schedule an appointment with their doctors.

## FACTS TO KNOW 5

### THE MEMORY CONNECTION

*Our immune system has an amazing strength—its amazing memory. It remembers every microbe it has ever fought and defeated. Immune system is a bit like artificial intelligence. We often think of our immune systems as reactionary, but the immune system is also designed to be preventative. Throughout your entire life, your body is exposed to a wide array of germs and bacteria. Each time your body is exposed to a new pathogen, it makes a record of the encounter. This memory of sorts allows the body to learn and adjust based on the new information it is provided about possible dangers. Most artificial intelligence systems learn in a similar manner: they're exposed to a situation, given prompts on what to do and then can address a similar situation in the future.*

*Vaccines introduce viruses that have already been killed or modified into the body. Our body doesn't know this, so it attacks, and thus, prepares the itself to stay safe in case the real virus ever invades.*

*There is an immune system disease called severe combined immunodeficiency (SCID), or 'bubble boy disease' that occurs in about 1 in every 100,000 births where a person is born with a deficient immune system, who must live out their life in a completely sterile environment because their body is unable to fight infections.*

*Skin is our first line of defence. It is made up of special cells that warn the body about incoming germs. The skin is also home to glands that can kill certain types of bacteria.*

*Our saliva and the tears in our eyes also have special chemicals that can break down many viruses and bacteria. Mucus in the nose, throat and lungs traps bacteria as well, and the acid in the stomach kills most germs.*

# V

## COVID-19 AND THE IMMUNITY QUESTION

# 31

# Beating COVID-19 and Its Collateral Damage

The fundamental factors for eating right, maintaining hygiene and leading a healthy, balanced life have always been important. However, they have become even more important in these corona-ridden times. COVID-19 took over our lives completely and has affected our mind and body extensively. Suddenly, every aspect of our way of living needs scrutiny and demands a complete overhaul, with the sole purpose of staying safe in these scary times.

The stress this virus added to our lives and the public health system of every country is unprecedented and devastating. What is clear is that certain lessons are best learnt quickly.

The most important lesson is to keep working on boosting our immunity continuously. We all need to keep doing our best to keep our immune systems strong to help our bodies fight not just COVID-19 but also many other mental and physiological issues that are cropping up because of it. Even though vaccines are now available, the best option before us is still prevention, and a strong immunity is an essential must-have to win this battle. We all need to focus on eating foods that boost our immune system and also make lifestyle choices (exercise, low stress, enough sleep) to ensure it.

The second lesson is to continue to follow the hygiene protocols strictly—maintaining strict social distancing, frequent hand washing, avoiding contact with our nose, mouth and eyes with contaminated hands, wearing a mask when stepping outside, using alcohol-based sanitizers, detecting and isolating infected people and avoiding unnecessary risks. Cleaning and sanitizing homes, offices and modes of transport regularly, washing vegetables and fruits thoroughly before using and sanitizing every store-bought commodity before getting it inside the house are important protocols to be followed. It is also important to avoid face-to-face meetings and restrict stepping out unless extremely unavoidable.

## Other Pitfalls of the Pandemic

Post COVID-19 our woes have not yet ended. Everyone is facing a different set of persistent symptoms. Besides the infection, which is extremely deadly, there are multiple other side effects of this pandemic that we need to look out for and tackle head-on before they cause a lot of damage.

### Fatigue

Fatigue is a common side effect that one faces during summer because of heat and dehydration. However, another factor, the omnipresent stress due to the pandemic is adding to it extensively. Also, it is prevalent among those who are suffering from COVID-19 or recovering from it. That is why it is essential to focus on food that can help combat it.

Simple steps help, such as easing the sugar intake, staying hydrated, adding more protein in the diet, cutting down on caffeine, eating magnesium-rich foods, having vitamin B12 and D supplements. Iron deficiency is also a common reason for fatigue, so focus on iron-rich foods like meats, organ meats, beans, chickpeas, nuts, seeds, whole grains and tofu.

## Anorexia

The constant need to try and eat healthy to boost immunity and the loneliness, stress and anxiety that everyone is facing as part of the package is leading to a silent rise of eating disorders among people of all ages.

Disordered eating for a long time can cause severe and lasting damage. If you suspect that you or someone you know might be suffering from an eating disorder, the sooner it is identified, the sooner it will be treated and the easier it will be for the person to recover.

## Weight Gain and Low Activity

Everyone seems to be facing this particular problem today. Lowered activity cannot be helped and as structured exercise such as going out for a walk or to the gym is out of the question, you need to increase your non-structured exercise.

Extra housework can help burn some extra calories; you can also add a few more activities (like washing the car or an hour of gardening) to keep your circulation going and also release some feel-good endorphins.

Following are some of the strategies that work:

- Play hide and seek with your children, engage in gardening, enrol in an online dance/aerobics/yoga class, or simply climb up and down the stairs.
- Eat only two regular meals and have fruits or vegetables for the third. This will help create a calorie deficit.
- Try out intermittent fasting—eat between an eight-hour window, let's say from 11.00 a.m. to 7.00 p.m. or 12.00 p.m. to 8.00 p.m. every day. Or do a weekly cleanse where you consume only fruits and vegetables.

- Make a rule not to eat in between meals and, if at all, then only fruits.
- Eat sweets just once a week.
- Similarly, eat fried foods just once a week.
- Drink enough water.

## Multiple Deficiencies

This is very common these days and care must be taken to add these important nutrients consciously in our diet.

- For calcium, include dairy, sesame (til) seeds and figs (anjeer) in your diet.
- For iron, have pomegranate, meats, lentils, chickpeas, gram flour (besan), etc.
- Eat enough fruits and vegetables to score a wide spectrum of vitamins and minerals.
- Sit out in the sun every day for some much-needed vitamin D.

## Constipation and Gut Troubles

Dehydration due to scorching heat in the summers and low water intake in the winters often encourages constipation. Additionally, almost nil exercise and restricted movement due to the frequent lockdowns (thanks to COVID-19), an overuse of medications (antacids are a common culprit, as they may cause the entire digestive system to back up, precipitating a vicious cycle that features heartburn and indigestion) and laxative abuse (these are habit-forming to the point where you need more and more until they simply stop working) are all factors that might lead to a constipation epidemic. So conscious steps must be taken to curtail it.

Fibre is the best solution and we need to consume 30–35 grams of fibre every day. While you are at it, get the right kind—insoluble fibre (also known as roughage) increases the feeling of fullness, stool size and bulk, and thus helps reduce constipation. Shun refined foods and zero in on whole foods, and consciously include more fruits and vegetables in your diet. Specific foods that work include okra, which besides constipation-fighting insoluble fibre is also loaded with vitamin B6 and folate; prunes, which are packed with natural laxatives (sorbitol and dihydrophenylisatin); and amla which stimulates the secretion of gastric juices and thus has a positive effect on digestion. Along with it, of course, you must drink enough water.

## Thyroid Damage

If you have been feeling unduly fatigued lately, are unable to cope and are suffering from insomnia, it is possible that your thyroid is acting up. It is time you go for a Thyroid Stimulating Syndrome (TSH) test, even if you consider yourself too young for thyroid disease and even if you are in the low-risk category.

The truth is that lockdown inactivity and continual stress and anxiety has been bad for our thyroid gland.

Here are a few things you can do:

- **Eat enough iodine**: This is an essential mineral for maintaining the functioning of the glands and healing them. So to prevent iodine deficiency, eat enough of iodine-rich foods like seaweeds, iodized salt and seafood.
- **Score enough selenium**: Selenium kickstarts the production of active thyroid hormones, so eat selenium rich foods like eggs, seafoods, organ meats, cereals and dairy products every day.
- **Get enough protein**: Besides its multiple other uses, protein is also important for the efficient working of

the thyroid gland. It is needed to transport the thyroid hormone to the tissues. Include dairy, eggs, nuts, seeds, lean meat, fish, nuts and seeds and legumes in your daily diet.

- **Keep the gut happy**: A well-functioning gut is important for the proper functioning of the thyroid gland, so include probiotics in your diet. Eat fermented foods, drink kanji, have homemade yoghurt often.
- **Zinc is important**: Zinc is a key nutrient for the thyroid and our body needs it to churn out the thyroid hormone. Too little zinc in the diet could lead to hypothyroidism. So, stock up on meats, seeds, dairy, eggs and whole grains.
- **Eat good fats**: Insufficient good fats in the diet can mess up all hormones, including thyroid. So, add flaxseeds, nuts, ghee, coconut and coconut oil to your diet.
- **Load up on antioxidants**: Foods that are high in antioxidants are also good for your thyroid. And berries are perfect for that. In fact, cranberries top the list in the ORAC scale, which ranks foods based on their antioxidant value. In fact, all fruits and vegetables deliver a good amount of antioxidants, so include them in the diet every day.
- **Things to avoid**: Avoid all forms of processed food, junk food, artificial sweeteners, BPA, chemical additives and too much sugar as these interfere with the thyroid function.

### Insomnia

To dramatically improve health and think clearly, be sure to get plenty of sleep. Unfortunately, sleeplessness has been on the rise and people of all ages are facing it these days. There are three reasons for it: first, the stress, frustration and anxiety, then there is the loss and grief that people have been facing for so long now, and third, lowered activity levels that do not tire us enough to be able to fall asleep quickly at night. This is bad news as prolonged sleep deprivation wears down our immune protection and thus weakens our ability to fight the infection.

---

## TO-DO:

- Be wary of too much caffeine late in the day (such as strong coffee late at night or cola and 'energy' drinks); it is a stimulant and can keep you awake when you actually want to drift to a cosy sleep.
- Try to eat foods that contribute to restful sleep—these are called sleepers. These are tryptophan-containing foods, an amino acid that the body uses to make serotonin that slows down nerve traffic, so your brain isn't so busy.
  - Dairy products such as cottage cheese, cheese, milk
  - Soy products such as soy milk, tofu, soybean nuts
  - Seafood
  - Meats
  - Poultry
  - Whole grains like bajra, barley, millets
  - Beans
  - Rice
  - Hummus
  - Lentils
  - Hazelnuts, Peanuts
  - Eggs
  - Sesame seeds, sunflower seeds

- Colocasia
- Sweet Potato
- Cashew nuts
- Mango
- Papaya
- Keep your dinner light; eat easily digestible foods. Khichri, a mixture of rice and lentils, is a wonderful sleep-inducing food.
- Haldi doodh is potent at inducing sleep. Add a pinch of pepper to ensure better absorption. Having a couple of walnuts at bedtime also helps.

---

## Heart Trouble

This pandemic has left our hearts weak in more ways than one. The level of stress, misery and loss unleashed by this pandemic weighed down heavily upon our hearts. The economic uncertainties caused a lot of distress. What's worse is that the after-effects of the infection continue to affect many people.

The COVID-19 infection, we now know, affects the inner surfaces of veins and arteries, which causes blood vessel inflammation, damage to very small vessels and blood clots in many people, affecting the heart and multiple other parts of the body as this compromises blood flow in the body. A lot of sudden cardiac arrests that happened later are now being attributed to this weakening of the system.

---

### TO-DO

First, going for regular screenings to detect cardiovascular damage are now even more important than earlier.

Second, extra weight definitely does not help your heart or your joints. It increases the workload on the heart and increases blood pressure—these have a detrimental effect on the heart. Work towards your ideal body weight. Monitor your body mass index (BMI) and keep it below 23.

Third, decrease risk and help heal the heart by exercising regularly. You can net the benefits even by walking for 30–45 minutes five times a week.

Finally, your diet needs to be overhauled with a clear focus on heart-healthy nutrition.

- Have a diet low in saturated fat, devoid of trans fats, and higher in monounsaturated fats. Put special emphasis on the consumption of omega-3 fatty acids. Vegetarians can get their dosage from flaxseeds, soy and mustard oils.
- Eat a diet low in simple carbohydrates; restrict refined flour foods, for example, biscuits, breads, naans, kulchas, cakes, pastries, mathris, other confectionaries and so on—all of which are part of Indian diet.
- Eat a diet high in dietary fibre. Increase the amount of vegetables and fruits that you consume.
- Cut down on sugar and salt intake as diabetes and hypertension are fast becoming an epidemic in India.
- If you are a non-vegetarian, try to include more fish in your diet. Eat lean meats.
- Eat 20–40 gm unsalted, non-fried nuts or seeds every day. These promote healthy lipid levels in the blood.

---

## Excess Hair Fall

COVID-19 and its side effects have left many of us weaker on the inside, with nutritional deficiencies, myriad health problems, hormonal changes, sudden weight loss (and then gain after recovery), unstable blood sugar, etc. It has affected our hair health drastically and replaced healthy hair growth with weakened hair shafts, frizzy, brittle ends, dull locks.

---

## TO-DO

Focus on these seven foods to regain your hair health:

- **Beetroot**: A vitamin B6 deficiency can cause reduced blood and oxygen supply to the hair, leading to hair loss, damaged hair and slow re-growth. Vitamin B6 also helps create melanin, the pigment that gives hair its colour. So, have beetroot for the essential vitamin.
- **Garlic**: Very often, hormonal imbalance shows up in the hair, particularly when the thyroid gland is involved. An underactive thyroid can result in frizzy or brittle hair while an overactive one can turn hair greasy and limp. Garlic helps to regulate the thyroid hormones because it supports blood-sugar metabolism (which is a big problem post COVID-19) and helps fight inflammation.
- **Pumpkin**: Yes, this humble food is very good for our hair and that's because it is loaded with vitamin A, which the body needs to promote the growth of the cells and tissues of the hair and scalp. Vitamin A also helps to produce healthy sebum (oil) in the scalp.
- **Eggs**: Protein is essential for every cell in the body, including those required for normal hair growth, particularly to replace the hair that has been shed. In fact, hair responds instantly to protein-rich foods. Eggs fit the bill as they are one of the best protein sources you can find. They also contain biotin and

vitamin B-12, which are important beauty nutrients.

- **Nuts**: Zinc is a mineral that helps in the maintenance of the oil-secreting glands that are attached to the hair follicles. Its deficiency can lead to hair shedding. Nuts, particularly cashews and almonds, are a terrific source of zinc, so make sure these nuts are a regular on your menu.
- **Amla**: A severe vitamin C deficiency can lead to hair-splitting and hair breakage as this antioxidant promotes hair cell growth and repair. Half an amla a day can help you meet your daily vitamin C requirements.
- **Water**: It helps to flush out the chemical wastes, toxins and other impurities from the body. It helps to transport the vitamins, minerals, amino acids and other nutrients in the body. So drink at least 8–10 glasses of water daily.

---

Finally, the most important rule is to focus on staying safe and in a positive mood. Eventually, this too shall pass. Till then, it is prudent to keep your head down, stay cheerful and continuously work on your health and immunity.

# 32

# Five Lessons to Learn from COVID-19

We have all gone through and are, in fact, still going through the difficult situation that the pandemic has unleashed on us. COVID-19 has been hard, and even though its reality and the challenges that it has brought up may be different for everyone, depending on their circumstance, there is absolutely no denying the fact that the only way forward from here is to learn from the pandemic to become a better, stronger, kinder and healthier person.

Here are some simple learnings that this debilitating, frustrating time has taught. These are lessons that can stand all of us in good stead, if we carry them forward consciously. These are spread across food, mind, lifestyle and are purely commonsensical. I am sure you will find them relatable.

## Lesson #1: Cook Frequently

Let's accept the fact: it is easy to just order in; so we succumb way too often. But you also know that it's not good for us. So, it is best to stick to fresh, safe home-cooked food.

Our consumption of restaurant meals and takeaways came down automatically during the lockdowns, thanks to their non-availability. After a few initial hiccups, we all managed fine, I believe.

We stuck to healthier home-cooked meals and that helped our health. We also realized that cooking is easier than we thought.

So going forward, let's make sure we cook more frequently at home and you'll definitely notice the difference, both on our wallet and weight.

Here are a few steps you can follow:

- Make a rule: Have a meal out (or order in) not more than twice a week.
- Invest in smart health gadgets. I find steamers, soup makers, sprout makers, rice cookers and kitchen scissors very helpful.
- Make a recipe book (you can make one on the computer or in your phone's Notes app) of no-cook and easy-to-cook recipes. Take a good look at your grandparents' cookbooks, call moms for recipes, ask friends, scour the Internet and put together a list of about 15–20 of these simple dishes that can be made in a jiffy.
- Learn to make one-pot recipes, which can be prepared putting all ingredients in a slow cooker. Meanwhile, complete your other chores or watch a movie. It'll be ready when you are back.
- Take an online cooking class and learn to cook some delicious and healthy foods if you have the time.
- Prepare in advance. Spend some part of the weekends, or an evening planning the weekly menu and preparing for it goes a long way.

## Lesson #2: Junk the Junk

Eating packaged junk food was on the rise during the lockdown because of multiple reasons—as a way of stress control, or because of their easy availability or simply to kill boredom and loneliness. This sustained wrong eating pattern can have big repercussions, and before one knows it, it has the potential to not just lead to weight gain, but also wreak havoc on the blood sugar and mess up the lipid profile by raising the bad cholesterol and triglycerides numbers.

Have you ever noticed that when you eat fried foods, you end up craving more? The fact is that cravings survive only when we continuously feed them. Cut them out with discipline and some innovative strategies and they will disappear.

Here are a few steps you can follow:

- Eat a healthy breakfast. This will take care of your cravings till lunch for sure. That's because insufficient breakfast (either in quantity or quality) sends a distress signal to your brain that triggers cravings.
- A substantial protein-rich lunch will take care of your cravings for the second half.
- Sometimes cravings scream of a nutritional deficiency. So, focus on eating a nutrient-loaded wholesome diet.

## Lesson #3: Practise Mindful Eating

Instead of succumbing to mindless eating in front of a screen or just gulping the tiffin down while working on a presentation, many people during the lockdown had the opportunity, the time and the possibility to have sit-down, non-hurried meals without any distractions. Try eating mindfully and see the difference, both in your health and soul.

I believe that this one change alone can help us lead a healthier, happier, disease-free life. Here are a few steps you can follow:

- Make eating meals together with family at fixed timings non-negotiable.
- Sit down and eat in a designated dining space.
- Focus on the food singularly. Keep the book closed, TV shut and your phone and laptop away from your dining table.
- Savour small bites and chew thoroughly. Food is meant to be savoured, not just eaten. This will also help you keep your portions in check and avoid overeating.

## Lesson #4: Stay Positive

Stress is a big killer. Chronic stress lowers the supply of killer immune cells that help our body fight infection and thus lower our immunity. Besides, stress and COVID-19 combined is a deadly combination. Times are tough due to the pandemic-induced stress, so staying positive is a tall order, but one that needs to be done hook or by crook.

Here are a few things you can do:

- Laugh some more because that can increase infection-fighting antibodies in the body, boost natural killer cells and lower immunosuppressive stress hormone cortisol. So, every day find something you can be happy about.
- Listen to music. This is an easy hack to boost your immunity (it soothes your soul). Even better than listening is making music. Go on, take some online tabla or guitar lessons for the sake of your immunity.
- Destress consciously. Find ways to destress that work for you, like reading a book, listening to music or meditating in the morning before you start your day

and at the end of the day. This twice-a-day ritual should help you stay fit.

## Lesson #5: Stay Prepared

It is important to continue to eat healthy, even in trying circumstances. In fact, more so in such circumstances of curtailed activity, lowered immunity and a sustained virus onslaught, it is smart eating that can help us stay healthy now.

Of course, there are challenges. Often there is only a limited set of available ingredients and storing and procuring a wide set of foods might be difficult (especially during lockdowns).

That said, there is still plenty that one can work with; all you need to do is to look closer in your kitchen cabinets and get a little more creative with the stuff at hand. The need of the hour is not just to score enough energy to last the day but also to derive the maximum nutrition possible from what we eat, while holding on to our sanity.

Here are a few steps you can follow:

- Learn how to use every last bit of the food you buy—the stem, the leaves, the peels, the fruit, the roots.
- Meal prep. Peel garlic, peel ginger, clean your coriander, arrange veggies in the fridge—put things that go bad front and centre (softer veggies) and the ones that last longer at the back of your fridge.
- Roast, steam or stir-fry veggies and store them in different boxes (pumpkin, sweet potato, brinjal, cauliflower, carrot, beans). Use them for salads or pastas or noodles or soup or as a side dish with grilled meats.

- Stock up boiled potatoes. It can help put together a dish—peas and potatoes, potatoes with yoghurt, potato salad, potatoes with beans, in a jiffy.
- Make some dishes that can be stored for later use, for example, tomato and coriander-mint chutney and onion gravy mix, so that you can use them as a curry base or sandwich spread quickly.
- Prepare for the next meal along with your first meal to save time.
- Recycle. When you cook, portion enough for two meals at least by giving them a makeover. Eat some, freeze some. This way you get a break from cooking sometimes and also have fewer dishes to wash when you reinvent with leftovers. For example:
  - Fry vegetables in a little oil and add some spices and leftover rice to turn them into scrumptious fried rice.
  - Turn leftover rotis into burritos.
  - Dry the leftover dal and make stuffed rotis or stuff them into sandwiches.
  - Lentils can come to your rescue every day. Just learn to use them creatively.
  - Boil some kidney beans (rajma), chickpeas (chana), black-eyed beans (lobiya) and keep them handy. In fact, one meal every day can be anyone of these lentils mixed with the already-prepped veggies, or just some quickly-chopped onions, cucumber and tomato.
  - Mix chickpea with boiled egg, cucumber and mayonnaise to make a salad.
  - Mash red kidney beans, combine with pizza seasoning and spread it on toast.

- ○ Thicken the masoor dal and mash into a 'pate' with grated crunchy vegetables or chopped onions.

# 33

# A Simple Post-COVID Diet Care Plan

COVID-19 has unfortunately touched the lives of many people. Even for those who have shaken off this virus after a miserable two weeks or so, the misery is slated to continue in many forms. Many COVID-19 survivors have been reeling under after-effects like headaches, chronic fatigue, difficulty breathing, joint pains, changes in taste and smell, medication-induced dry mouth, brain fog, sleep issues and multiple more such symptoms which have been lingering for a long time, sometimes as long as five to six months. Any of these issues suffered for a certain amount of time can severely impact our quality of life.

Here is a post-COVID-19 diet care plan that can help you.

## Hydrate Yourself

Our body loses a lot of fluids during infection, so your priority should be to replace that loss. Drink plenty of water to speed up your recovery. Target drinking eight to 10 glasses of water every day. Try to include other hydrating drinks like flavoured water, soups, broths, green teas and non-caffeinated beverages in your daily diet.

## Focus on Protein

A high-protein diet is essential as protein can help repair the damaged body tissues and make up for the lost muscle mass during the infection. Also, enough protein in the diet is important to keep the immunity in good shape and save you from further diseases. Focus on lentils, legumes, nuts, dairy, eggs, white meat, soy and fish. Try to score at least 1 gram protein per kilogram of body weight every day. For example, if you weigh 60 kilograms, ensure that you consume at least 60 grams of protein every day. You can even increase it to 1.5 gram protein per kilogram of body weight for a few days. Make sure you include one to two portions of protein in every meal and have two protein-rich snacks every day.

Besides quantity, it is important to focus on the quality of protein too. Try to eat complete proteins that deliver all the essential amino acids. Most non-vegetarian sources are complete proteins, but if you are a vegetarian, then a judicious combination like, dal and rice or roti and dal can give you complete protein.

## Focus on the Gut

COVID-19 tends to leave the gut in a terrible shape, leading to multiple gastric issues. The medicines also play havoc with the gut microbiome, killing the good bacteria. So, it's our responsibility to rebuild and rebalance the bacteria in the gut painstakingly. Focus on eating probiotic food daily. Include at least one fermented food in your daily diet—homemade yoghurt, sprouts, dhokla, sourdough bread, kanji, kimchi, etc. If the gut is in bad shape, a course of probiotic tablets will help restore the balance of good and bad bacteria.

## Eat Easily Digestible Food

It is best to stick to home-cooked food to recover fast. This will give your digestive system a break and let the body speed up the recovery process. Eat dishes like khichri, poha, simple subzis, raita, etc., and avoid fried, rich fare entirely for a few weeks.

## Skip Dieting

This is not the time to try and lose weight or go for a calorie deficit. Let the body recover first. More calories will deliver more energy to the body to fight off the infections and help it heal faster and regain strength. So, opt for healthy but calorie-dense foods.

## Focus on Wholesome Nutrition

COVID-19 stresses the body extensively and the multiple medicines debilitate your body. Consciously include foods rich in vitamin A, E and minerals like zinc and magnesium to help the body heal better and build immunity.

## Work on Your Memory

The virus is known to damage the memory cells, which is why brain fog is a symptom of COVID-19. In order to regain the lost attention, cognitive thinking abilities and memory, focus on iron which you can get from extra-lean red meat, beans, peas, dark green leafy vegetables, pomegranate and dried apricots; omega-3, in fatty fish, walnuts, flaxseeds; monounsaturated fatty acids, primarily present in vegetable oils and particularly extra virgin olive oil; vitamin B which is found in dairy, eggs, dark green leafy vegetables; and astaxanthin, a form of microalgae. To score astaxanthin, eat plenty of salmon, algae (seaweeds, spirulina) and shellfish (shrimp, prawn, crab, lobster). There is, unfortunately, no known vegetarian source yet.

## Boost Your Mood

COVID-19 is a major happiness sucker too. It leaves everyone dealing with anxiety and blues. So, it helps to tailor the diet accordingly. There are clearly some happy nutrients and happy foods that can positively affect our mood and should be included in your diet. My top seven picks are: turmeric, chickpeas, walnuts, apples, pumpkin seeds, dried figs and bananas as they all are loaded with compounds that boost happiness. Eat at least two of these every day.

# V

## TOOLS

# 34

# 50 Immunity Boosters

Our immune system is powerful, but it needs help every now and then and this is where the immunity boosters come into play. They work in multiple ways:

- They strengthen the body's disease fighting forces and keep the body battle ready and primed for destroying any invader that comes its way.
- They increase the number of immune cells and make them more aggressive and effective.
- They slow down and combat the production of free radicals that cause a lot of damage in the body.
- They enhance communication within the immune cells, thus making them more efficient.
- Years of exposure to stress and oxidants takes its toll on the immune system. They keep the strength of the body up by mitigating the damage.

## Foods That Help

**Immunity Booster #1**

Flaxseeds have been revered for ages and for a good reason. They contain alpha-linolenic acid, omega-3 fatty acid and phytoestrogens called lignans—all these ingredients are important in modulating the response of our immune system. Sprinkle flaxseeds on your breakfast or just add to your dals.

**Immunity Booster #2**

Include carrots in your diet. Bugs Bunny rarely came down with the flu, because of a good reason. Carrots, his food of choice, contain loads of beta carotene, which gets converted into vitamin A in the body, a powerful phytonutrient that boosts the immune system's production of infection-fighting natural killer cells and T-cells. It also contains vitamin B6 which boosts the production of antibodies. Carrot pudding, anyone? Or just have carrot sticks dipped in dressing or blended in a veggie juice.

**Immunity Booster #3**

Munching on fresh jamuns during summer season was a given earlier. Not so much anymore, unfortunately. But it is time to begin snacking on it again as there is a good amount of vitamin C and other antioxidants in this fruit, which can help stimulate the production of WBCs and boost our immune system.

**Immunity Booster #4**

Barley has disappeared from our kitchens, but it needs to make a comeback. It contains beta-glucan, a type of fibre with potent antimicrobial and antioxidant capabilities. It boosts immunity, speeds wound healing and also helps antibiotics work better. It has selenium too, a difficult to find trace mineral that has a powerful positive effect on our immune system.

**Immunity Booster #5**

In the time before chips and sodas, sweet and sour chickpeas (khatte cholle) was a delicacy everyone looked forward to at least twice a week. That's because they deliver a lot of antioxidants and zinc, which help to control inflammation in the body. Zinc deficiency is, in fact, linked to lowered immunity, as it plays an important role in the function of the T-cells, natural killer cells and lymphocytes, which are some of the power houses of our immune system. Try to have half a cup of cooked chickpeas (alternating between them) thrice a week at least.

### Immunity Booster #6

There's a reason why sweet potato chaat was so popular earlier. It is high in vitamin C, which is a brilliant antioxidant and also delivers vitamins A and E—a dynamic duo for immune-system boosting and is full of fibre.

### Immunity Booster #7

Mushrooms were probably not a part of our traditional food platter, but it makes sense to include it now. They are a rare food source of vitamin D, which is essential for good immunity. Also, they increase the production of cytokines in the body, the cells that help fight off infection. They contain polysaccharides, which are compounds that support the immune system, and also help with the production of WBCs in the body.

They even deliver selenium, glutathione and ergothioneine—all known to function as antioxidants and are rich in fibre (good for gut health). So make it mandatory to have mushroom soup twice a week, add them to all stir-fries, even to your meat dishes.

### Immunity Booster #8

Have at least two servings a week of fatty seafood, such as sardines, salmon, herring and mackerel for your omega-3 fatty acid fix. If you are a vegetarian, have other foods like walnuts and flaxseed to boost the immune system.

**Immunity Booster #9**

Pumpkin helps. In addition to beta carotene (vitamin A), pumpkin delivers vitamin C, vitamin E, iron and folate—all of which strengthen the immune system. So more pumpkin in your diet can help your immune cells work better to ward off germs and speed healing.

**Immunity Booster #10**

Go nuts (and seeds):

- Pumpkin seeds: This power food is rich in protein, iron, zinc and phosphorus, as well as the essential fatty acids needed to keep your immune system functioning well.
- Sunflower seeds: Studies show vitamin E, a powerful antioxidant, fights respiratory infections, including cold. It boosts the responses of antibodies and certain immune system cells when we're under stress—and who isn't? A quarter cup of sunflower seeds has almost all the vitamin E you need daily.
- Almonds: A quarter cup of almonds provides 50 per cent of your Vitamin E requirement. Brazil nuts pack a whopping dose of selenium, a mineral that also boosts wintertime defences.
- Try seeds toasted and sprinkled over salads, or combine them with dried fruit for a power snack. Instead of chips or cheese noodles for an afternoon snack, reach for a handful of nuts or seeds.

### Immunity Booster #11

Eat raw onions and green chillies with all meals. This is a perfect way to stay protected from infections. Both of them contain powerful flavonoids that have antibiotic and immunity-boosting effects. To score more benefits, cut open the onion and let it sit for about 10 minutes to increase the phytonutrient content.

### Immunity Booster #12

If you want to boost your immune system efficiently, adding some spinach regularly to your diet is a great place to start. Spinach contains vitamin K, folic acid and calcium. Besides boosting eye health and lowering blood pressure, it also helps fight oxidative stress and thus boosts immunity.

### Immunity Booster #13

Phytonutrients found in honey have antibacterial and antiviral properties that can help boost the immune system. Honey is also loaded with both enzymes and minerals, which help strengthen immunity. You can have raw honey, or mix it in lemon water, warm water, green tea or even kaadha. You can also drizzle it over oats, yoghurt, etc. Honey's high nutrient density makes it an amazing energy booster too.

## Eat Right

### Immunity Booster #14

Eat an immunity boosting breakfast. It is tempting to skip breakfast as there is just too much to do in the mornings, and many think that missing this meal means extra time gained.

However, by missing this very important meal, not only do

you start on the wrong foot, run the risk of lowered stamina and brain fog, but also prime yourself for gaining some weight. Breakfast skippers get more cravings through the day and end up piling the pounds.

That's not all. Not many know that breakfast is a brilliant opportunity to include some immunity boosting foods and nutrients in your diet.

So, you must include:

- Whole grain to score vitamin B
- A citrus fruit or amla shot for vitamin C
- An antioxidant loaded vegetable like sautéed spinach or mushrooms or carrots
- A complete protein like eggs or yoghurt
- Good fats like seeds or nuts
- A hot mug of ginger tea to score epigallocatechin gallate (EGCG), an antioxidant that fights viruses effectively

**Immunity Booster #15**

Focus on vitamin B12 and avoid its deficiency. Those with vitamin B12 deficiency tend to have suppressed natural killer cells activity and decreased number of circulating lymphocytes.

**Immunity Booster #16**

Incorporate immunity building foods into your diet in the form of fermented food and beverages. These foods are rich in vitamin C, zinc and iron that aid in boosting the immunity. There's also a link between gut health and immunity. The better your gut, the better your immunity. Fermented foods and beverages improve digestion, help restore the balance of friendly bacteria.

Other positives are mental health, weight loss and heart health.

### Immunity Booster #17

Write down the names of five richly coloured vegetables and fruits that you really like, then add to the list two vegetables that you're curious about and are willing to try. Now assign one to each day from Monday to Saturday and make sure you have it on that day, every week.

This will add the much-needed fibre and detoxifying mineral and vitamins to your diet which are chock-full of phytonutrients, protein, vitamins and antioxidants.

## Drink Right

### Immunity Booster #18

Dehydration is very often the reason for lowered immunity and, of course, a myriad of other health problems. So, stay hydrated. This can boost your immune health immensely. Water helps the body produce lymph, which carries WBCs and other immune system cells. So, drink enough water, every day. In fact, begin the day with water first thing in the morning. Also try eating more hydrating foods like cucumbers, melons, spinach, oranges, etc.

### Immunity Booster #19

Your grandma was right—hot chicken soup is perfect to clear clogged airways and keep the immunity high. This nourishing broth provides solid nutrition, prevents dehydration and replaces lost salt from the body, besides keeping the body warm from within and so, it is extremely conducive to our immunity.

## Immunity Booster #20

Start drinking warm water with a squeeze of lemon juice and honey first thing in the morning.

It'll cleanse out the toxins from the body and help your organs work efficiently. Besides, it has major anti-fungal, immunity-boosting and detoxification properties. Lemon juice is also nature's best tool for aiding digestion, destroying bacteria and cleansing the system. This is the ideal drink for restoring acid-alkali balance in the gut and maintaining the body's internal 'climate' at a pH which supports healthy bacteria instead of the viruses and harmful bacteria that thrive in more acidic environments. Remember how your grandpa used to begin his day with this simple but wondrous drink? Now you know why!

## Immunity Booster #21

Green tea is packed full of antioxidants as well as flavonoids which fight off harmful bacteria. It is also an excellent relaxation tool which offers one of the best ways to fight off an infection, as our immune system is suppressed when you are down and depressed. It also delivers EGCG which is found in green tea and has powerful and proven antioxidant benefits.

## Herbal Heroes

## Immunity Booster #22

Dry ginger powder, also known as sonth, is a ground form of dried ginger roots. It is a traditional spice that is eaten more in winters as it is warming. It is not just a taste enhancer, but also contains essential oils and multiple immunity-enhancing vitamins like beta carotene, vitamin C, B and minerals like potassium, calcium, zinc, iron and copper. So, add a pinch to all your dals, just blend it in warm water and sip, or make ginger tea with it.

**Immunity Booster #23**

Have giloy (heart-leaved moonseed). This lesser-known medicinal herb delivers calcium, phosphorus, iron, copper, zinc and manganese and is loaded with antioxidants. It is a known immunity booster and sugar level stabilizer. Just squeeze the leaves and mix it with amla juice and drink. Or mix the powder with warm water and have it.

**Immunity Booster #24**

Oregano is a powerful antibacterial and anti-fungal herb, thanks to the presence of powerful compounds called phenols—carvacrol and thymol. It is a powerful antioxidant, is anti-inflammatory, a natural antibiotic and pain killer, protects against toxins and supports the immune system. So, sprinkle oregano liberally on your food.

**Immunity Booster #25**

Onion seeds (kalonji) contain an essential ingredient, thymoquinone, that helps to fight against the inflammation that builds up within the lungs due to pollution or infection. It is a potent mood booster too.

Sprinkle onion seeds liberally on dal, vegetables and even chapatti to get the benefit. Or have cold pressed kalonji oil.

**Immunity Booster #26**

You may already know this that ginger is known to help with nausea. It also has anti-inflammatory benefits and contains vitamins that help fight infections. An ingredient packed with immune-boosting benefits, ginger also helps prevent nausea and soothes an upset tummy. Ginger is also very effective in keeping your body warm and helps break down the accumulation of toxins in your organs. Add ginger to a stir-fried dish or boil it to make a cup of ginger tea with some added lemon for a pleasant and a healing hot drink.

**Immunity Booster #27**

With its antiseptic, anti-fungal and nutritive properties, garlic has been used as an immune booster for thousands of years by Ayurveda. It is a powerful natural antioxidant, which protects the body from bacterial and viral infections, without causing any side effects. Garlic acts as a natural antibacterial agent when it is fresh and raw as it contains allicin that kills viruses and bacteria. It is a good medicine against coughs, colds and chest infection during winter. Swallow a lightly crushed garlic clove with a glass of water first thing in the morning every day.

**Immunity Booster #28**

Eat more dal. A lentils-based diet delivers more arginine—an amino acid that's been shown to increase both carbohydrate and fat burning—besides improving the immunity immensely and controlling blood pressure. Make sure you eat a variety of dal. There are so many dals to choose from, eat them all by rotation. And opt for unpolished lentils to score maximum nutrition.

**Immunity Booster #29**

Eat the apple with the peel. Apple is rich in quercetin, the compound that improves lung function and helps beat most modern-day lifestyle diseases. Check this comparison: apples without skin contain less than half the amount of quercetin as whole apples, and its juice has about less than one-tenth the amount. So, keep the peel to keep your lungs strong and general immunity up, especially looking at the way pollution is taking over our lives these days. Just wash it thoroughly before eating.

**Immunity Booster #30**

Trust ghee. Ghee is a good source of highly beneficial butyrate, a short-chain fatty acid that acts as a detoxifier, improves colon health, aids digestion, improves insulin sensitivity and boosts our immunity too.

## Lifestyle Tips

**Immunity Booster #31**

However busy you might be, please sit in the afternoon sunlight for 15 minutes every day at least. But, why do you need the sun?

The answer is simple. It is a scientifically proven solution to get enough vitamin D. Sun rays help our body make vitamin D, an essential vitamin that helps boost our immunity immensely. They also keep our spirits up and blues away. The best news is that getting some sun every day is a thing that can be very easily done.

**Immunity Booster #32**

Step out in natural light. Besides helping the body make vitamin D, sunlight also helps the skin cells produce a very powerful immune-boosting substance called interleukin-1 (IL-1). So that morning walk or sipping your morning tea sitting in the balcony can actually help boost your immunity.

### Immunity Booster #33

Oral hygiene is important for our immunity too. That is why it is important to pay extra attention to our toothbrush.

If you share a bathroom with others, be sure your toothbrush doesn't come into contact with other toothbrushes. Viruses can easily spread if it comes in contact with other brushes or an unhygienic surface. Though basic, it is an important advice.

Keep it in an upright holder so it can dry properly. Also, replace your toothbrush if you have been sick, to start fresh.

### Immunity Booster #34

If you have stepped out, quickly wash your hands, especially before eating or touching your face. Also, to completely kill the bacteria that causes infection, wash them thoroughly with soap and warm water, then dry them properly too.

## Mind Power

### Immunity Booster #35

Deep breathe before you begin eating a meal. This helps the body get into the rest and digest mode, and powerful belly breaths actually help activate the primary nerve that influences digestion. Do this for a few days, before every meal, and you will notice a huge difference in your gut health. And better gut health translates into stronger immunity.

### Immunity Booster #36

Practise compassion. It is directly connected to improving our immune system and stimulating the pro-social networks in your brain and reducing loneliness. All these help enhance the immunity.

**Immunity Booster #37**

Do you...

- tend to worry a lot about myriad things?
- take care of other people more than yourself?

You should know that chronic stress downs the supply of killer immune cells (help our bodies fight infection) which translates to a lowered immunity.

We have approximately 60,000–80,000 thoughts a day, most of them being repetitive and negative. These negative thoughts lead to small releases of cortisol all day long in the body, and this unrelenting influx constantly keeps suppressing our immune system, making us sitting ducks for the invaders out there waiting to harm us.

But you can't stop thinking, can you? So, the solution in this case is to tame your worries and put a lid on stress:

- Practise pausing. Feel a destabilizing emotion like fear or worry taking over your mind? Consciously extricate yourself from the process, take a conscious pause and make an effort to observe the situation and how you are reacting to it from a third person point of view. This detached observation will let you look at the situation without judgement and stay aloof from it.
- Calm your mind consciously. Breathe slowly and deeply; reach a certain level of calm and only then dissect the oppressive emotion, as if looking from the outside. This way your response will be more balanced.

## Immunity Booster #38

Do forest bathing. Spending time in the greens is a very effective way to jumpstart our immunity. There is solid science behind this.

Firstly, our genes are designed to respond positively to fresh air and a green environment.

Secondly, when we spend time in nature, we breathe in molecules called phytoncides. These antimicrobial organic compounds derived from plants get into our bloodstream and boost our overall health and immunity. They are known to boost our happiness, reduce the stress hormones, lower the heart rate and blood pressure, up our immune system and also hasten recovery from illness.

So, make sure you take out time to sit next to your plants, or in a nearby park every day, as your life may practically depend on this simple ritual.

## Immunity Booster #39

Put writing to use. Writing is therapeutic, especially for our immune system. When you write down your feelings, fears, anxiety and thoughts, it helps the body release tension and thus heal better. It is a very useful tool and has been found to bust stress, improve sleep, reduce autoimmune diseases like rheumatoid arthritis and also boost the immunity response by upping the levels of T lymphocyte immune cells. It also supports the release of distressing emotions that could otherwise suppress immune function. So, commit to regular journaling or write about specific emotional events that bother you.

## Immunity Booster #40

Meditate every day. Meditation effectively sends a signal to our body that there isn't a stress storm coming after us and that we are safe. It calms both the mind and body, and this helps lower inflammation, strengthen the immune response. Meditation can be as simple as sitting still in a quiet place, and then working at quietening the thoughts in the mind. Chanting a mantra or an affirmation repeatedly works very effectively too. And you can do this for as little as five to 10 minutes at a time.

**Immunity Booster #41**

Let those tears flow. Here's why: deep sobs open the chest and diaphragm, releasing bound-up energy. This helps to free your heart of muscular tension. A good cry also enhances oxygen delivery to the cells and stimulates release of specific neurochemicals in the brain that promote relaxation.

**Immunity Booster #42**

Laugh some more. Our first line of defence against any disease is happiness. A real belly laugh increases infection-fighting antibodies and boosts the activity of natural killer cells. Yes, watching a comedy or an online stand-up show can actually up our immune system's response. What's more, it seems that just anticipating a humorous encounter can enhance immunity too. This happens because laughter lowers stress hormone cortisol levels and thereby protects our immune system. So, look around and find stuff that you can be happy or cheerful about, or better still really laugh about. And do this constantly. Force yourself to smile and laugh as much as you can.

**Immunity Booster #43**

Listening to music can boost your immunity as long as it is music that you like and music that soothes your soul. It has been found that listening to music that sends shivers down the spine or that gives people chills stimulate the same 'feel-good' parts of the brain that good food and sex activate and raise the levels of immunoglobulin A (IgA), a protein from the immune system that helps fight infections. So, listen to your favourite tunes and listen often.

### Immunity Booster #44

Make some music. There's something even better than listening to music, and that's making it. For example, a drumming session has been found to lead to greatly enhanced natural killer-cell activity afterwards. So go on take some weekend drum or guitar lessons—all for the sake of your health. In addition, playing a musical instrument has been shown to lower cortisol, stress, anxiety and depression, all of which down our immunity.

What better excuse to dust off your guitar, drums, or finally learn to play the piano?

### Immunity Booster #45

Do you want an immunity-boosting secret? Keep your friends close. Social support and camaraderie of friends can be good medicine. Our immune system likes it when we spend time with friends. So, feed friendships to starve colds. A regular nightout with your pals is healthy and so, no more guilt on that!

## Things To Avoid

Finally, we come to a section on what to avoid, steps that can inadvertently boost our immunity.

### Immunity Booster #46

Drink responsibly. Excessive alcohol intake can harm the

body's immune system in two ways. First, it leads to an overall nutritional deficiency as it interferes with the absorption of nutrients in the body, particularly vitamins B1, B3, folate and vitamin A and also prevent the body from fully absorbing and using zinc, iron, calcium and folic acid. This leads to a shortage of all critical immunity-boosting nutrients in the body. Second, alcohol also reduces the ability of white cells to kill germs. Damage to the immune system increases in proportion to the quantity of alcohol consumed. So, watch how much you drink.

## Immunity Booster #47

Don't over medicate. Not only can drugs become addictive, but every single drug has a negative side-affect. Some medicines like aspirin, beta blockers, antacids, anti-inflammatory, anti-ulcer and diabetes-control drugs can decrease the body's ability to absorb vitamins (particularly D, A, C, E and B12).

Antibiotics disturb the bacterial flora in the intestine (kill the good bacteria that help with digestion), which also affect absorption of nutrients from the food we eat. Similarly, long-term use of contraceptive pills may deplete three B vitamins—folic acid, B12 and B6, as well as zinc and magnesium. So, keep a check on the medicines that you take.

## Immunity Booster #48

Don't go overboard with your supplements. Large doses of vitamins and minerals are not only completely unnecessary, but also carry certain risks. Excessive levels of zinc, for example, can disrupt the body's uptake of copper, a known immunity booster itself. Vitamin D without adequate level of magnesium does not get metabolized properly, and in high doses, it can be toxic.

Some herbal supplements can also interact with prescription medications. So, stick to food as they contain a wide range of vitamins, minerals and antioxidants that work in synergy to protect your health.

## Immunity Booster #49

Tannins in tea hinder the absorption of iron and zinc from foods and caffeine in coffee reduces our body's ability to absorb dietary calcium and also increases its excretion via the kidneys. So drink these beverages at least half an hour before/after your meals, and take your iron and calcium supplements too two hours before/after your cuppa.

## Immunity Booster #50

Don't follow starvation or restrictive diets. Similar to how your car needs petrol to run, your body needs enough nutrition to function properly. It needs nutrients to keep all the systems functioning, including our immune system. The immune system is made up of cells and proteins that defend against infection. To make these essential components, your body needs energy, which comes from the food and drinks you put in your body. So never starve as that's the easiest way to invite an infection to come over and take hold.

# 35

# 25 Super Easy Immunity Hacks

1. Eat raw garlic every morning and add it liberally while cooking.
2. Drink at least one cup of green tea every day.
3. Eat cruciferous vegetables (kale, broccoli, cauliflower, cabbage) in your diet at least three to four times a week.
4. Eat raw onions and green chillies with every meal.
5. Eat soya beans or tofu two to three times a week.
6. Exercise for 30 minutes five times a week.
7. Meditate for 10 minutes every day.
8. Say a prayer before meals.
9. Write in a journal or diary every day.
10. Use turmeric and other spices liberally in cooking.
11. Practise deep breathing for a few minutes every day.
12. Eat one type of whole grain (by rotation) at least once every day.
13. Eat leafy greens at least once every day.
14. Eat shiitake or reishi mushrooms two times a week.
15. Include one root vegetable such as carrot, turnip, sweet potato, yam, beets in your daily diet.
16. Eat beans or lentils at least five times a week.
17. Eat fish two to three times a week.
18. Drink ginger tea at least once a day.
19. Have one tbsp roasted seeds every day.

20. Eat two to three servings of different colour fruits every day.
21. Speak to one good friend every day, even if for just a few minutes.
22. Be tolerant and practise forgiveness.
23. Take a warm bath; it calms, relaxes the muscles and improves circulation.
24. Fast once or twice a week.
25. Include some raw food (fruits and vegetables) in your daily diet.

# 36

# RECIPES

Immunity-Boosting Dishes

**Cooling Cucumber Dip**

Grate a cucumber. Finely chop up four garlic cloves and few fresh mint leaves. Juice a lemon. Add all the ingredients in a bowl and stir to combine. Refrigerate for an hour before digging in. Enjoy this dip with baby carrots, celery or any other vegetable of your choice. It's refreshing, light on the stomach, immunity-boosting and super delicious.

**The benefit:** You score multiple antioxidants, lots of hydration and vitamin C.

**Avocado and Balsamic Vinegar Sourdough Toast**

Remove and discard the peel and pit from an avocado. Place the avocado in a small bowl and add salt, pepper to taste, and 1 tbsp lemon juice. Mash the mixture lightly with a fork to combine. Toast your sourdough bread—top toasted bread with avocado mixture. Add thinly sliced tomato and sprinkle some red pepper flakes. Garnish with basil leaves and a drizzle of balsamic vinegar.

**The benefit:** You score multiple minerals, vitamins A, C and E, and loads of good fats from the avocado. Sourdough bread is fermented and so it is good for the gut.

## Cold Pumpkin Salad

Cut half a pumpkin into small cubes and steam them. Dice an apple (don't peel) and cut few leaves of lettuce into strips. Finely julienne some ginger and combine it with the rest of ingredients for the dressing.

Toss the pumpkin, apple and lettuce in a bowl and drizzle the dressing on top.

**The benefit:** You score lots of vitamin A from the pumpkin and lots of quercetin from the apple.

## Buckwheat Noodles

Boil 100 grams of buckwheat noodles in the broth of your choice or water. Season the broth with salt and pepper according to taste. Dice 100 grams of shiitake mushrooms and add to the noodle pot. Once the noodles are soft, add 100 grams of seasonal greens—I like to use spinach.

**The benefit:** Mushrooms deliver antioxidants and are a rare food source of vitamin D. Buckwheat is gluten-free and easier to digest.

## Kidney Beans (or Black-Eyed Peas) Bruschetta

In a pot, add water, salt and 50 grams of kidney beans or black-eyed peas. Boil till the beans are cooked. Drain the excess water. Transfer the cooked beans to a bowl and mash lightly. Leave some beans whole for a varying texture. Combine the beans with 50 gram of yoghurt, rosemary and mustard. Season with salt and pepper to taste. Finely dice some tomato, lettuce and cucumber. Toast the multigrain bread on both sides till it's brown and crunchy. Add the prepared mixture and layer the fresh vegetables on top of the mixture. Drizzle some extra virgin olive oil on top. Enjoy as a hearty breakfast or snack.

**The benefit**: Beans deliver lots of soluble fibre and nutrients and rye bread again is very rich in fibre.

### Brown Rice Salad

Cook 30 grams of brown rice in salted boiling water. Finely chop the spring onion and dice the red pepper. In a pan over low to medium heat roast some cashews and sunflower seeds on low heat, till brown and fragrant.

For the dressing, finely mince a few garlic cloves and whisk together with a drizzle of oil, a teaspoon of soy sauce and the juice of a lemon. Add salt and pepper to taste.

Once the rice is cooked, transfer it to a bowl while still warm, combine with a chopped spring onion, red pepper, roasted cashews and sunflower seeds and toss well.

Transfer the salad to a serving dish and drizzle the dressing on top.

**The benefit**: Brown rice delivers fibre, vegetable antioxidants, and cashews and seeds deliver many hard-to-find trace minerals that are important for our immune system.

### Cold Sweet Potato Salad

Peel and dice two sweet potatoes and one apple into half-inch cubes. Boil the sweet potatoes until tender. Once the pan is off the heat and cooled to room temperature, refrigerate for a few hours. Meanwhile, to a blender, add olive oil, cilantro, chopped green onions, lemon juice, mustard paste, garlic and black pepper and pulse a few times.

Add chopped apples and the cooled sweet potatoes to a salad bowl and toss. Season with salt and pepper to taste.

Drizzle the dressing on the salad and garnish with green onions.

Refrigerate for an hour and enjoy!

## Mashed Sweet Potatoes

Roughly chop two sweet potatoes and boil till tender. Drain the water and to the steaming pot add butter and mash the potatoes. Ensure that no lumps remain. Add cinnamon, nutmeg and honey to the pot and combine.

Serve as a tasty and healthy side dish to your favourite meal.

**The benefit**: Both deliver lots of potassium, vitamin C, B vitamins, anthocyanin, beta carotene and fibre.

## Chickpeas and Fruit Salad

Wash and dice an apple into cubes. Mix gently with boiled ½ cup chickpeas and ¼ cup pomegranate seeds. Make a dressing by mixing extra virgin olive oil, red wine vinegar, freshly crushed pepper. Add salt to taste.

Pour over salad and mix gently so that chickpeas and fruits are coated well with the dressing.

## Hummus

Soak ½ cup chickpeas in water overnight. Pressure-cook till they are soft and can be mashed easily between your fingers.

To a mixer, add the cooked chickpeas, 1 tbsp sesame paste, few crushed garlic cloves, lemon juice, olive oil and salt to taste. Blend till smooth.

**The benefit**: Chickpeas are packed with antioxidants—vitamin C, E and beta carotene, and have loads of mineral manganese too.

## Beetroot Salad

Dice two beetroots into cubes and boil. For the tempering, heat up ghee in a ladle and add cumin seeds, curry leaves and chopped green chillies. Once the tempering begins to sputter, remove from the heat. Add the tempering to 1 cup yoghurt along with the ginger paste and salt to taste. To the yoghurt mix, add the beetroot and combine well. Garnish with mint leaves.

**The benefit**: Beetroot delivers compound betaine that triggers glutathione s-transferase (GST) activity, which is important for the elimination of toxins and cleanse our body.

## Immunity-Booster Drinks

### Drink 1: Herbal Help

Boil few fresh holy basil (tulsi) leaves, carom seeds, cumin seeds, mango powder, salt (one tsp each) and few mint leaves in water for 10–15 minutes. Sip it warm or at room temperature.

**The benefit**: This drink helps to prevent dehydration and it is well known that dehydration can down our immunity extensively.

### Drink 2: Lemon–Ginger–Green Tea Infusion

Grate some fresh ginger into a pot of water and boil. Add in some green tea and brew for a few minutes then strain.

Add few slices of lemon, let the water cool to room temperature and then refrigerate.

**The benefit:** Lemons are a great source of vitamin C, which is known to boost the immune system, prevent disease, fight the common cold and protect cells; ginger adds multiple antioxidants that are protective too.

### Drink 3: Amla Juice

Blend two chopped amla with water. Filter and discard the pulp. Add pepper and a few drops of honey (optional).

**The benefit:** Amla is the richest natural source of immunity-boosting vitamin C.

### Drink 4: Flaxseed Churn

Beat one cup yoghurt till smooth. Add 1 tbsp roasted flaxseeds and a fruit of choice and combine.

**The benefit:** Flaxseeds contain alpha-linolenic acid, omega-3 fatty acid and phytoestrogens called lignans—all these ingredients are important in modulating the response of our immune system.

### Drink 5: Amla, Carrot and Lemon Juice

Juice the powerful trio of 1 amla, 3–4 carrots and one lemon and sip fresh.

**The benefit:** Carrots deliver beta carotene, amla gives vitamin C and lemons help restore the acid-alkali balance in the body, all three forming important immunity-strengthening steps.

# Acknowledgements

I want to thank a lot of people, but I will begin by thanking all the editors I have worked with across different media houses. The list is really long and I am indebted to each one of them for everything they have taught me. I was so raw when I began and they have helped shape my writing and made it and me better with each successive stint. Some of them are such dear, dear friends today and I love and cherish them all.

The entire team at Rupa, my editor, Yamini, for her support and advice, Saswati for editing the book so brilliantly again, and of course, my publisher, Kapish, for continuing to have faith in my ideas.

To my agent, Anuj Bahri, Redink for relentlessly championing my writing and showcasing my books so brilliantly.

All my friends who love me and encourage me selflessly—I love you back and more.

My husband Bhanu, my son Vimanyu, who are my world.

My sister Punita and her family for just being there for me all the time.

And of course, as always, my parents, whom I love and respect immensely.